Social Disparities in Thoracic Surgery

Editor

CHERIE P. ERKMEN

THORACIC SURGERY CLINICS

www.thoracic.theclinics.com

Consulting Editor
VIRGINIA R. LITLE

February 2022 • Volume 32 • Number 1

ELSEVIER

1600 John F. Kennedy Boulevard ● Suite 1800 ● Philadelphia, Pennsylvania, 19103-2899

http://www.thoracic.theclinics.com

THORACIC SURGERY CLINICS Volume 32, Number 1
February 2022 ISSN 1547-4127, ISBN-13: 978-0-323-91959-3

Editor: John Vassallo (j.vassallo@elsevier.com)
Developmental Editor: Jessica Nicole B. Cañaberal

Thoracic Surgery Clinics (ISSN 1547-4127) is published quarterly by Elsevier Inc., 360 Park Avenue South, New York, NY 10010-1710. Months of publication are February, May, August, and November. Business and editorial offices: 1600 John F. Kennedy Boulevard, Suite 1800, Philadelphia, PA 19103-2899. Periodicals postage paid at New York, NY, and additional mailing offices. Subscription prices are $405.00 per year (US individuals), $875.00 per year (US institutions), $100.00 per year (US students), $473.00 per year (Canadian individuals), $893.00 per year (Canadian institutions), $100.00 per year (Canadian students), $225.00 per year (international students), $494.00 per year (international individuals), and $893.00 per year (international institutions). Foreign air speed delivery is included in all Clinics' subscription prices. All prices are subject to change without notice. **POSTMASTER:** Send address changes to Thoracic Surgery Clinics, Elsevier Health Sciences Division, Subscription Customer Service, 3251 Riverport Lane, Maryland Heights, MO 63043. **Customer Service (orders, claims, online, change of address): Telephone: 1-800-654-2452 (U.S. and Canada); 314-447-8871 (outside U.S. and Canada). Fax: 314-447-8029. E-mail: journalscustomerservice-usa@elsevier.com (for print support); journalsonlinesupport-usa@elsevier.com (for online support).**

Reprints. For copies of 100 or more, of articles in this publication, please contact Commercial Rights Department, Elsevier Inc., 360 Park Avenue South, New York, NY 10010-1710. Tel: 212-633-3874; Fax: 212-633-3820; E-mail: reprints@elsevier.com.

Thoracic Surgery Clinics is covered in *MEDLINE/PubMed (Index Medicus), EMBASE/Excerpta Medica, Science Citation Index Expanded (SciSearch®), Journal Citation Reports/Science Edition,* and *Current Contents®/Clinical Medicine.*

Contributors

CONSULTING EDITOR

VIRGINIA R. LITLE, MD
Section Chief of Thoracic Surgery,
Cardiovascular Surgery, Medical Director of
Thoracic Surgery, Intermountain Healthcare,
Murray, Utah

EDITOR

CHERIE P. ERKMEN, MD
Professor of Thoracic Surgery, Program
Director, ACGME Thoracic Surgery Fellowship,
Program Director, Lung Cancer Screening,
Professor, Center for Asian Health, Temple
University Health Systems, Lewis Katz School
of Medicine at Temple University, Philadelphia,
Pennsylvania

AUTHORS

SAKIB M. ADNAN, MD
Resident, Department of Surgery, Einstein
Healthcare Network, Philadelphia,
Pennsylvania

MARA B. ANTONOFF, MD
Associate Professor, Department of Thoracic
and Cardiovascular Surgery, University of Texas
MD Anderson Cancer Center, Houston, Texas

LEAH BACKHUS, MD, MPH
Department of Cardiothoracic Surgery,
Stanford University, Stanford, California

IAN C. BOSTOCK, MD, MSc
Fellow in Cardiothoracic Surgery, Department
of Thoracic and Cardiovascular Surgery,
University of Texas MD Anderson Cancer
Center, Houston, Texas

DUYKHANH P. CEPPA, MD
Associate Professor of Surgery, Associate Vice
Chair of Professional Development, Diversity,
and Wellness, Division of Cardiothoracic
Surgery, Indiana University School of
Medicine, Indianapolis, Indiana

DAVID T. COOKE, MD, FACS
Associate Professor, Chief, Division of General
Thoracic Surgery, Department of Surgery,
University of California, Davis Health,
Sacramento, California

IRMINA ELLIOTT, MD
Department of Cardiothoracic Surgery,
Stanford University, Stanford,
California

LORETTA ERHUNMWUNSEE, MD, FACS
City of Hope Comprehensive Cancer Center,
Duarte, California

CHERIE P. ERKMEN, MD
Professor of Thoracic Surgery, Program
Director, ACGME Thoracic Surgery
Fellowship, Program Director, Lung
Cancer Screening, Professor, Center for
Asian Health, Temple University Health
Systems, Lewis Katz School of Medicine
at Temple University, Philadelphia,
Pennsylvania

JAIRO ESPINOSA, MD
Department of Thoracic Surgery, Temple
University, Philadelphia, Pennsylvania

LUIS A. GODOY, MD
Assistant Professor, Diversity and Inclusion
Director, Division of General Thoracic
Surgery, Department of Surgery, University of
California, Davis Health, Sacramento,
California

CAYO GONZALEZ, BA
Department of Cardiothoracic Surgery,
Stanford University, Stanford, California

**RIAN M. HASSON CHARLES, MD, MPH,
FACS**
Dartmouth-Hitchcock Medical Center Geisel
School of Medicine at Dartmouth, Lebanon,
New Hampshire

ELISE HILL, MD
General Surgery Resident, Department of
Surgery, University of California, Davis Health,
Sacramento, California

LARRY R. KAISER, MD, FACS
Managing Director, Alvarez & Marsal, New
York, New York; Adjunct Professor of Surgery,
University of Pennsylvania Perelman School of
Medicine, Philadelphia, Pennsylvania

VIRGINIA R. LITLE, MD
Section Chief of Thoracic Surgery,
Cardiovascular Surgery, Medical Director of
Thoracic Surgery, Intermountain Healthcare,
Murray, Utah, USA

NATALIE LUI, MD
Department of Cardiothoracic Surgery,
Stanford University, Stanford, California

JESSICA MAGARINOS, MD
Department of Surgery, Temple University
Health Systems, Department of General
Surgery, Temple University Hospital,
Philadelphia, Pennsylvania

KYLE G. MITCHELL, MD, MSc
Resident in General and Cardiothoracic
Surgery (4+3), Department of Thoracic and
Cardiovascular Surgery, University of Texas
MD Anderson Cancer Center, Houston, Texas

MUHAMMAD FARHAN NADEEM, MD
Cardiothoracic Surgery Fellow, Temple
University Hospital, Philadelphia,
Pennsylvania

KEITH NAUNHEIM, MD
St. Louis School of Medicine, St Louis,
Missouri

MEGHNA PATEL, BS
City of Hope Comprehensive Cancer Center,
Duarte, California

TAKSHAKA PATEL, MD
Department of Surgery, Temple University
Health Systems, Department of General
Surgery, Temple University Hospital,
Philadelphia, Pennsylvania

ALLAN PICKENS, MD
Associate Professor of Surgery, Emory
University, Atlanta, Georgia

MICHAEL POULSON, MD
Resident, Department of Surgery, Boston
Medical Center, Boston University School of
Medicine, Boston, Massachusetts

VARUN PURI, MD, MSCI
Division of Cardiothoracic Surgery,
Washington University School of Medicine, St
Louis, Missouri

SIVA RAJA, MD, PhD, FACS
Associate professor of Surgery at Lerner
College of Medicine at the Case Western
Reserve University, Surgical Director,
Center for Esophageal Diseases,
Cleveland Clinic Foundation, Cleveland,
Ohio

VIGNESH RAMAN, MD, MHS
Resident, Surgery, Duke University School of
Medicine, Durham, North Carolina

SIMRAN K. RANDHAWA, MD
Division of Cardiothoracic Surgery, University
of Colorado School of Medicine, Aurora,
Colorado

SOPHIA H. ROBERTS, MD
Department of Surgery, Washington University
School of Medicine, St Louis, Missouri

ERNESTO SOSA, MSW, MPH
City of Hope Comprehensive Cancer Center,
Duarte, California

JASON STRUNK, DO
Department of Surgery, Inspira
Health Network, Vineland,
New Jersey

BETTY C. TONG, MD, MHS
Associate Professor of Surgery, Cardiovascular
and Thoracic Surgery, Duke University School
of Medicine, Durham, North Carolina

VALEDA YONG, MD
Resident, Surgery, Temple University Hospital,
Philadelphia, Pennsylvania

Contents

Social disparities in lung cancer diagnosis, treatment, and survival have been studied using national databases, statewide registries, and institution-level data. Some disparities emerge consistently, such as lower adherence to treatment guidelines and worse survival by race and socioeconomic status, whereas other disparities are less well studied. A critical appraisal of current data is essential to increasing equity in lung cancer care.

The many socioeconomic disparities in the myriad of diagnoses that make up benign lung diseases are unfortunately a global issue that was most recently highlighted by the COVID-19 pandemic of 2020. In this chapter, we will be reviewing the socioeconomic disparities in benign lung disease from both a United States perspective as well as a global perspective. We will cover the spectrum of infectious, obstructive, and restrictive lung disease and review the evidence on how social disparities affect these populations and their access to medical care.

Since the initial report of long-term survival after lung transplantation (LT) in 1983, there has been remarkable progress in the field and LT is now the gold-standard therapy for patients with end-stage lung disease. It confers a significant survival advantage and improves the quality of life in patients who often have few other treatment options. However, LT remains a complex undertaking and establishing and maintaining an LT program is resource intensive with multiple potential barriers. In this article, we focus on disparities in LT and the potential solutions to improving access to LT.

Esophageal cancer is a deadly cancer. Advances in multimodal treatment have improved esophageal cancer outcomes. Advancements have not benefited all races equally. Major disparities in esophageal cancer outcomes exist. Minorities undergo fewer surgical resections of esophageal cancer and have poorer outcomes.

Research on health disparities in thoracic surgery is based on large population-based studies, which is associated with certain biases. Several methodological challenges are associated with these biases and warrant review and attention. The lack of standardized definitions in health disparities research requires clarification for study design strategy. Further inconsistencies remain when considering data sources and collection methods. These inconsistencies pose challenges for accurate and standardized downstream data analysis and interpretation. These sources of bias should be considered when establishing the infrastructure of health disparities research in thoracic surgery, which is in its infancy and requires further development.

THORACIC SURGERY CLINICS

SERIES OF RELATED INTEREST

Advances in Surgery
http://www.advancessurgery.com/

Surgical Clinics
http://www.surgical.theclinics.com/

Surgical Oncology Clinics
https://www.surgonc.theclinics.com/

THE CLINICS ARE AVAILABLE ONLINE!
Access your subscription at:
www.theclinics.com

Foreword
Social Disparities in Thoracic Surgery: Actionable Items

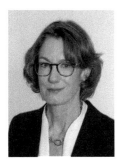

Virginia R. Litle, MD
Consulting Editor

We are excited to bring you this focused issue for the *Thoracic Surgery Clinics* on "Social Disparities in Thoracic Surgery." An established expert on this topic, Dr Cherie Erkmen, our guest editor, created a primer for how to address disparities not only in the management of lung cancer screening (LCS) but also in designing health disparities research projects, diversifying our thoracic surgery workforce, and working to level the playing field in health care delivery. Thanks to the novel coronavirus pandemic, these have become timely subjects, and the energy to make a difference is palpable not only in our clinical arena but also in our daily extracurricular life. Every day on social media (#SoMe) and in the press we read about examples of social and health care disparities from police brutality to inequity in vaccine distribution. As surgeons, we are integral components of society. Our mission is to care for people. But also, as surgeons we like action and are accustomed to using a rulebook to accomplish our goals. The content of this issue provides guidance with actionable items. Example: how do you address disparities in LCS or esophagectomy rates? You educate primary care physicians about the LCS guidelines. You establish a centralized LCS program to unburden the workload of primary care physicians. You acknowledge that implicit bias has affected race-related differences in the patient-physician relationship, and then you provide unconscious bias training to your team so they can deliberately change. How do we optimize health care delivery? You can run for office and write your US senators and members of Congress; however, a more grass-roots approach includes supporting access to telehealth through your system and connecting with community leaders to address cultural challenges and the distrust in the health care system. Thank you to our outstanding contributors and thanks to the earnest effort of Dr Erkmen for providing a thorough compendium of socially relevant content for thoracic surgeons. Think globally and act locally.

Sincerely,

Virginia R. Litle, MD
Section of Thoracic Surgery
Cardiovascular Surgery
Intermountain Healthcare
5169 So. Cottonwood Street, Suite 640
Murray, UT84107, USA

E-mail address:
virginia.litle@imail.org

Twitter: @vlitlemd (V.R. Litle)

1547-4127/21/© 2021 Published by Elsevier Inc.

Preface

First Steps in Addressing Health Disparities in Thoracic Surgery

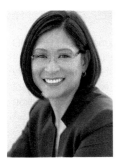

Cherie P. Erkmen, MD

Editor

In the constitution of the World Health Organization, health is defined as "one of the fundamental rights of every human being without distinction of race, religion, political belief, economic or social condition."[1] The COVID-19 worldwide pandemic demonstrated that health is very much a function of all these factors. We can empirically measure differences in health outcomes and mortality. However, to address root causes and develop interventions to correct health disparities, we must delve deeper into mechanisms. We must scrutinize biased assumptions, discriminatory actions, and a failure to act.

Firmly held traditions may impede our path to health equity. For example, we in the thoracic surgery community widely accept race correction of spirometry results. Race correction originated from scholarly work of Thomas Jefferson and a contemporary physician named Samuel Cartwright. They asserted innate, biological differences between races, specifically, pulmonary "deficiency in the Negro" of "20 percent." Furthermore, they used these assumptions to justify

slavery by concluding that forced labor invigorates "the red vital blood sent to the brain that liberates their minds when under the white man's control, and it is the want of sufficiency of red vital blood that chains their minds to ignorance and barbarism when in freedom."[2,3] In present-day evaluations, spirometry software automatically invokes a correction of 10% decrease for black patients and 6% decrease for Asian patients[4] once race is entered.[5] If we pause to think about the implications of this, we assume that non-white patients have less "vital capacity" than white patients. If we assume race impacts pulmonary function, how do we consider environmental, social, economic, educational, employment, and other factors in this calculation? Or, are we using race as an oversimplified proxy for all these factors? From a utilitarian standpoint, how should we correct for people of mixed race or races other than black and white? Is race a biologic difference or social construct? Are disparate outcomes a biologic difference and/or a result of access to quality care?

Thorac Surg Clin 32 (2022) xiii–xiv
https://doi.org/10.1016/j.thorsurg.2021.10.001
1547-4127/22/© 2021 Published by Elsevier Inc.

As overwhelming as these questions are, our focus should be on achieving health equity. Health equity does not mean that everybody receives the same treatment, nor does it mean that everyone is expected to have the same outcome. Health equity is striving to reach each individual's highest potential of health. In this landmark work, we begin to develop a framework for answering these questions of health disparity within thoracic surgery. We look at the historical context of health policy and health care delivery in the United States (articles by Magarinos and colleagues and Nadeem and Kaiser), health disparities with specific disease process within our practice (articles by Raman and colleagues, Elliott and colleagues, Espinosa and Raja, Randhawa and colleagues, and Pickens), how study design, enrollment, and data management impact our approach to health disparity (articles by Adnan and colleagues, Charles and colleagues, and Mitchell and colleagues), and how disparities in thoracic training and workforce impact health disparities (Ceppa and Godoy and colleagues).

The past few years have prompted many of us to see structural racism, sexism, and discrimination. Culturing a curiosity allows us evaluate problems objectively, to "think more deeply and rationally."[6] Diverse curiosity, or "curiosity associated with the interest in exploring unfamiliar topics and learning something new," is associated with quality problem-solving and originality.[7,8] Understanding and addressing health disparities in our practice demand this first step of curiosity. We should try to avoid divisive shame or blame, but instead question mechanistic underpinnings of health disparity. Unfortunately, we have seen a backlash against exploration of structural discrimination. It has been disparaged as "woke" or "cancel" culture. Being curious is not a political stance; it is the foundation of empathy and innovation, which is desperately needed in the field of health disparities.

This issue represents innovation from the contributors, who have analyzed current evidence with a fresh perspective. I would like to thank the authors, who have exceeded all expectations to deliver something new to thoracic surgery. I am indebted to John Vassallo for his enthusiastic support, and the staff at Elsevier, especially Jessica Cañaberal, who has been a skilled and consummate professional. I am most grateful to Virginia Litle for having the courage and vision to conceive a health disparities issue of *Thoracic Surgery Clinics*. It has been one of the greatest honors of my career to be entrusted with this meaningful endeavor at this critical time.

Cherie P. Erkmen, MD
Temple University Health Systems
Temple University Hospital–Thoracic Surgery
3401 North Broad Street
Suite C-105, Parkinson Pavilion
Philadelphia, PA 19140, USA

E-mail address:
cherie.p.erkmen@gmail.com

REFERENCES

1. Available at: https://www.who.int/about/governance/constitution. Accessed.
2. Cartwright S. Report on the diseases and physical peculiarities of the Negro race. New Orleans Med Surg J 1851;7:691–715.
3. Cartwright S. Slavery in the light of ethnology. In: Elliott E, editor. Cotton is king and proslavery arguments. Augusta, GA: Abbott & Loomis; 1860.
4. Lujan HL, DiCarlo SE. Science reflects history as society influences science: brief history of "race," "race correction," and the spirometer. Adv Physiol Educ 2018;42(2):163–5 PMID: 29616572.
5. Braun L. Race, ethnicity and lung function: a brief history. Can J Respir Ther 2015;51(4):99–101.
6. Available at: https://hbr.org/2018/09/the-business-case-for-curiosity. Accessed.
7. Hardy JH III, Ness AM, Mecca J. Outside the box: epistemic curiosity as a predictor of creative problem solving and creative performance. Pers Individ Diff 2017;104:230–7.
8. Available at: https://today.oregonstate.edu/archives/2016/nov/curiosity-can-predict-employees%E2%80%99-ability-creatively-solve-problems-research-shows. Accessed.

A History of Health Policy and Health Disparity

Jessica Magarinos, MD[a,b], Takshaka Patel, MD[a,b], Jason Strunk, DO[c], Keith Naunheim, MD[d], Cherie P. Erkmen, MD[e,f],*

KEYWORDS

• Health care disparities • Health care policy • Health care legislation • Medicaid • Medicare
• Health care in US

KEY POINTS

- The history of health care policy demonstrates structural inequities that contribute to health disparities in the United States.
- Although US Congress has debated universal health care coverage for almost 100 years, the first major, comprehensive policy was passed in 1965 to establish Medicare and Medicaid.
- With Medicare and Medicaid being the only national health policies, people in the United States relied on employee-based health plans, private insurance, or no insurance, leading 48 million uninsured or underinsured people in 2010.
- The Affordable Care Act aimed to provide a comprehensive plan through a combination of increased eligibility for Medicaid, Medicare, and subsidized private insurance.
- Despite legislation, US Supreme Court rulings, Presidential Executive orders, and government agencies addressing health care, disparity of access, care, morbidity and mortality impacts marginalized populations.

Health policy is a relatively broad term meant to encompass a government decision or plan of action to address health needs such as access, delivery, quality, and efficiency. Health policy affects every citizen through every stage of life. Other parties intrinsically invested in health policy include health care professionals, hospital and health systems, private and government health organizations, pharmaceutical companies, health care product companies, and insurers. The National Health Expenditure of the United States is $3.8 trillion, which represents 17.7% of the gross domestic product and growing at a rate of 5.4% annually.[1] Health policy at the federal, state, and local levels significantly impact not only everyone's individual health status but also the current state of health disparities. This work summarizes landmark health policies and how they have shaped the unique health care environment in the United States (**Fig. 1**). To understand health disparities, we must learn the history of the current infrastructure. To mitigate further health disparities, we must leverage all relevant resources including health policy.[2,3]

The Declaration of Independence defines unalienable rights of life, liberty, and the pursuit of happiness. The Bill of Rights defined Amendments to the US Constitution, specifically addressing

[a] Department of Surgery, Temple University Health Systems, 3401 N. Broad, Parkinson Pavilion, Suite C405, Philadelphia, PA 19140, USA; [b] Department of General Surgery, Temple University Hospital, 3401 N. Broad, Parkinson Pavilion, Suite C405, Philadelphia, PA 19140, USA; [c] Department of Surgery, Inspira Health Network, Vineland, NJ, USA; [d] St. Louis School of Medicine, St Louis, MO, USA; [e] Center for Asian Health, Lewis Katz School of Medicine at Temple University Hospital, 3401 N. Broad Street, Suite 501, Parkinson Pavilion, Philadelphia, PA 19140, USA; [f] Department of Thoracic Medicine and Surgery, Temple University Health Systems, 3401 N. Broad Street, Suite 501, Parkinson Pavilion, Philadelphia, PA 19140, USA

* Corresponding author. Lewis Katz School of Medicine at Temple University, Temple University Health Systems, 3401 N. Broad Street, Suite 501, Parkinson Pavilion, Philadelphia, PA 19140.
E-mail address: Cherie.erkmen@tuhs.temple.edu

Thorac Surg Clin 32 (2022) 1–11
https://doi.org/10.1016/j.thorsurg.2021.09.013

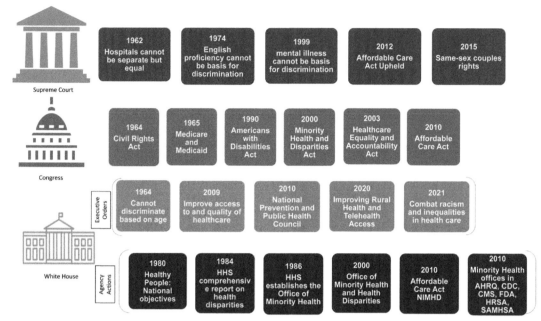

Fig. 1. Landmark actions of the US Supreme Court, Congress, and Presidency. Health and Human Services (HHS), National Institute of Minority and Health Disparities (NIMHD), Agency for Healthcare Research and Quality (AHRQ), Centers for Disease Control and Prevention (CDC), Centers for Medicare & Medicaid Services (CMS), Food and Drug Administration (FDA), Health Resources and Services Administration (HRSA), and the Substance Abuse and Mental Health Services Administration (SAMHSA).

protection of individual citizens and limitation of the US Government. However, in 1857, the US Supreme Court ruled that the unalienable rights did not apply to free or enslaved Black Americans because they were not citizens when the Constitution was written (*Dred Scott v. Sanford*). Eight years later in 1865, the US Congress passed and states ratified the Thirteenth Amendment making slavery unlawful and granting the US Congress the power to enforce protection of freedom. The Fourteenth Amendment defined "All persons born or naturalized in the United States are citizens. . . [none shall] deprive any person of life, liberty, or property, without due process of law; nor deny to any person within its jurisdiction the equal protection of the laws." The Fifteenth Amendment specifically names the right to vote regardless of "race, color or previous condition of servitude." Although Amendments XIII through XV protect civil rights of individuals in general, they do not specifically include health. Dr Martin Luther King explained that, "Of all forms of inequality, injustice in health is the most shocking and inhuman because it often results in physical death."

LANDMARK LAWS AND US COURT DECISIONS

Landmark laws and US Court decisions have played a major role in shaping health and health

disparity. Constitutional Amendments XIII through XI defined citizens of the United States with rights and privileges and gave the US Congress power to uphold these privileges. However, the US Supreme Court upheld the notion that public resources could be equal but separate (*Plessy v. Ferguson* [1896]). Another 50 years would pass before the interpretation of equitable rights would be challenged successfully. The Supreme court ruled that enforcement of exclusive housing covenants was unconstitutional (*Shelley v. Kraemer* [1948]) and separate but equal education was unconstitutional (*Brown v. Board of Education* [1954]).

The issue of separate but equal came to health care in *Simkins v. Cone* (1963).[4] George Simkin, a dentist and National Association for the Advancement of Colored People (NAACP) leader joined African American physicians and filed suit against two North Carolina hospitals. The suit claimed that these hospitals denied "admission of physicians and dentists to hospital staff privileges, and the admission of patients to hospital facilities, on the basis of race." The US Supreme Court defined hospitals receiving federal funding as arms of the state and thus subject to constitutional guarantee of equal protection. Furthermore, separate but equal in the setting of hospitals was deemed unconstitutional.

These landmark US Supreme Court Rulings set the context for the Civil Rights Act of 1964; specifically, Title VI prevented discrimination based on race, color, or national origin by government agencies that receive federal funds.[5] The *Lau v Nichols 1974* ruling asserted the language could not be used as a proxy of discrimination on origin; entities receiving federal funds cannot discriminate based on English proficiency. The Americans with Disabilities Act of 1990 established rights for individuals with disabilities, focusing on integrating those with disabilities to all rights and privileges of citizenship. The *Olmstead v. LC 1999* ruling asserted that mental illness was a form of disability, and that the isolation of those with mental illness was a form of discrimination.[6] Similarly, *Obergefell v Hodges (2015)* upheld that same sex marriage was a fundamental right with the privileges of marriage, which include access to health insurance.[7]

The first comprehensive law to address the link between marginalized populations and health disparity was passed in 2000. Edward Kennedy sponsored the Minority Health and Disparities Act that appropriated support "for research, training, dissemination of information, and other programs with respect to minority health conditions and other populations with health disparities." It also established the National Center on Minority Health and Health Disparities within the National Institutes of Health. This center eventually evolved to the National Institute on Minority Health and Disparities (NIMHD) with the Affordable Care Act (ACA). In 2003, Representative Elijah Cummings and 125 US Representatives sponsored the Healthcare Equality and Accountability Act. The purpose of this Act is to "improve minority health and health care and to eliminate racial and ethnic disparities in health and healthcare." This Act was groundbreaking in addressing coverage of undocumented legal immigrants under Medicaid and State Children's Health Insurance Program and directs the Health and Human Services to pilot, a project for migrant workers. It also calls to improve health care for those with limited English proficiency and specific provisions for Native Americans. Representative Jesus Garcia and 106 cosponsors have introduced the Health Equity and Accountability Act of 2020, which provides for technology programs to collect and interpret health disparities data, support health workforce diversity, and increase access to culturally and linguistically appropriate health care. The most controversial portion of the proposal attempts to reduce health disparities among noncitizens through modification of eligibility of Medicare, Medicaid, private health insurance and other programs.

The Civil Rights Act and sequent laws and rulings addressed longstanding de facto (in practice) and de jure (in law) discrimination. Though these were milestones in reversing de jure discrimination, they are limited in addressing de facto discrimination, especially as it relates to health care. Robust mechanisms to prevent, monitor, and penalize discrimination in health and health care were not developed. To date, the Office of Civil Rights under the US Department is Education is the major enforcement agency for preserving equity in health including the Civil Rights Act of 1964, Age Discrimination Act of 1975, Public Health Service Act, Americans with Disability Act, and the Affordable Care Act.[8,9]

MEDICARE

The idea of government-assisted health care coverage for American citizens can be traced back to President Franklin D. Roosevelt's new deal during the Great Depression. Many variations of universal health care were introduced to the United States Congress in the years following the New Deal. However, without bipartisan support, a nationally funded healthcare system was never passed into law. The concept of focusing on the elderly became a strategy for increasing the chances of passing a bill. Retired Americans and those older than 65 years often did not have the means to obtain employer-provided health insurance. This older population also had greater health care needs than other age groups. Additionally, they were a population that heavily participated in voting and exercised influence among lawmakers. President John F. Kennedy advocated for a program that could aid the above 65 retired population, which became known as Medicare. After his assassination, President Lynden B. Johnson and a democratic majority in congress carried forth the Medicare initiative.

On July 30, 1965, Medicare was first passed into law as The Social Security Amendments of 1965. At this time, Medicare was sectioned into Part A and Part B. Part A included mandatory hospital stay coverage for all persons aged greater than 65. Part B included voluntary additional outpatient physician visit coverage for all persons aged greater than 65.

From the beginning, Medicare implementation played an important role in desegregation. Title VI in the Civil Rights Act of 1964 stated that federal funds could not be allocated or utilized at segregating institutions, and the Johnson administration ensured Medicare funds would not be an exception. Eager for Medicare payments, hospitals around the country quickly desegregated, marking an important positive milestone in the Civil Rights Movement as well as health equity.

The limits of Medicare implementation were tested shortly after its conception. In 1969, the Gottschalk Report demonstrated success of hemodialysis for end-stage renal disease. Media coverage and popular support of hemodialysis as a treatment option for end-stage renal disease prompted Congress to pass the Social Security Amendments of 1972.[10] This amendment expanded the population eligible for Medicare to include persons under 65 who were diagnosed with end-stage renal disease. The Social Security Amendments of 1972 also added coverage for persons younger than 65 who had been receiving Social Security Disability payments for 24 months. Like those with end-stage renal disease, those with 24 months of demonstrated disabilities had advanced and costly health care needs without a means to pay for them. However, many disabled individuals may be too sick or disabled to survive the 24-month wait period. The 24-month wait period is a policy that neglected people who could benefit from intervention.[11]

Other gaps in Medicare coverage came to light upon implementation, including mostly dental, vision, hearing, and long-term care, as well as care outside of the United States. Additionally, copays for 20% of costs and deductibles can rapidly mount with any serious or chronic condition. There is no limitation on the maximum out-of-pocket expense. These gaps in coverage and limitless expenses disproportionately affect those in lower income strata.[12] About 40% of low-income beneficiaries spent 20% or more of their incomes on out-of-pocket expenditures for premiums and medical care. This disproportionate burden not only limits access to health care among low-income families, but also forces them to choose between health care and other necessities of living.

To address gaps of coverage, Medicare Part C, now known as Medicare Advantage, was passed as part of the Tax Equity and Fiscal Responsibility Act (TEFRA) (Medicare at 50) Medicare Advantage allows for risk-based, private health plans to contract with Medicare and Medicare enrollees.[13] Beneficiaries pay supplemental premiums to a private Medicare Advantage plan and in turn receive health insurance for all services. The private Medicare Advantage plan receives a predetermined, monthly, risk-adjusted payment from the Medicare program to cover each beneficiary's care. In 2021, 42% of Medicare beneficiaries enrolled in Medicare Advantage plans.[14] Unfortunately, minorities and those with low socioeconomic status are less likely to enroll in Medicare Advantage or supplemental insurance.[15] Though Medicare Advantage and other supplemental insurances were designed to address the gaps in basic Medicare coverage, premiums and cost-sharing of these plans has disproportionately excluded minorities and underserved populations from affordable care. Furthermore, understanding the infrastructure of Medicare and its multiple parts, enrollment, and the utilization of benefits can be challenging for all Medicare patients, but even more so in those with low health literacy, mistrust in health care, and/or language barriers.[16]

Low participation in Medicare Advantage and supplemental insurance translates into decreased utilization of preventive care and office visits and increased utilization of costly emergency room and hospital visits among marginalized populations. Possibly, policies that invest in equity in access to preventive and routine health care may improve population health and decrease overall health care costs.

In 1988, The Medicare Catastrophic Coverage Act added prescription drug coverage to attempt to reconcile a noted large defect in Medicare coverage. However, prescription drug coverage was later repealed in The Omnibus Budget Reconciliation Act of 1989 due to growing frustrations regarding the increasing Medicare premiums. The frustrations seemed to stem primarily from the higher socioeconomic status Medicare beneficiaries who were already enrolled in supplemental insurance or were the recipient of retirement insurance from their previous employer. Meanwhile, primarily the lower socioeconomic status beneficiaries benefited from the additional Medicare coverage because they did not typically have other sources of coverage. As a result, the higher socioeconomic status population strongly opposed the increase in premiums they were faced with and had enough voting power to overturn the previous decision.17 In 2003, under President Bush and the Republican party, after a growing need for assistance with prescription drug payments, The Medicare Modernization Act reintroduced prescription drug coverage, known as Part D.[16,17]

The Medicare Improvements for Patients and Providers Act of 2008 ensured coverage for preventative services met the recommendations of the US Preventative Services Task Force (USPSTF). The National Lung Screening Trial published in 2011 demonstrated annual low-dose computed tomography screening instead of chest radiograph (LDCT) screening decreased lung cancer mortality by approximately 20%. Resultantly, the USPSTF recommended annual LDCT screening for all individuals aged 55 to 80 with a history of more than 30 pack-years of smoking. The Centers for Medicare and Medicaid Services approved ILDCT screening in patients 55 to 77 years old with a history of than 30 pack-years of smoking and who are current smokers or quit within the past 15 years.[18]

MEDICAID

The Social Security Amendments of 1965 created Medicaid, a program designed to supplement state medical coverage to persons who already met welfare requirements. Medicaid was conceived by Representative Wilbur Mills who had opposed government-funded health care coverage. It is believed he created Medicaid so further discussions about broadening to universal health care coverage could not use the poor population as a bargaining tool. That would explain the significantly looser regulation of Medicaid and lack of structure when compared with its counterpart, Medicare. The initial covered population included the populations that were already eligible for government welfare payments: single parent households, the elderly, the blind, and the disabled. Medicaid eligibility was also allotted to children in double-parent households below a certain income threshold (known as Ribicoff children) and anyone the states deemed to be medically needy but did not meet the income requirement.[19]

The Social Security Amendments of 1967 introduced the Early and Periodic Screening, Diagnostic, and Treatment Program (EPSDT) aimed to provide routine care to children in response to an emergence of research documenting the long lasting negative physical and psychological effects on disadvantaged poor children who were neglected by the health care system.[20] The Social Security Amendments of 1972 allowed states to further expand their coverage to include beneficiaries younger than 22 years of age hospitalized in a psychiatric facility. The Omnibus Budget Reconciliation Act of 1986 extended coverage to include all pregnant women and children up to 100% of poverty, which was further expanding in the following few years to a higher poverty cutoff. The Omnibus Budget Reconciliation Act of 1990 introduced a Medicaid-funded prescription drug monetary assistance program.

Medicaid was initially conceptualized as a state-based program with federal funding and as such has been largely variable dependent on the state. Medicaid initially required states to provide coverage to all interested persons who were at or below the set poverty level or fell into one of the following defined at-risk populations: disabled,

blind, children, pregnant women, and the elderly. Initially, the states were also required to pay sufficiently for health care services so that care would not be affected. Starting in 1981, several waivers were issued to individual states, relieving them from strictly following all preset Medicaid guidelines and granting them more flexibility with how to utilize the funding. Most notably, the 2005 Deficit Reduction Act (DRA) granted states permission to provide "benchmark coverage" instead of ensuring services provided through Medicaid coverage. Additionally, cost-sharing of 10% to 20% of medical expenses, previously prohibited, were now permissible up to 5% of a family's income.[21] States can also limit Medicaid benefits to households at more than 150% of the poverty level ($39,750 for a household of 4).[22] Critics of the DRA assert that the implementation of cost-sharing, limited coverage, and premiums may make health care inaccessible for the exact population Medicaid is designed to protect. Proponents of the DRA prioritize the need to contain health care costs and that increasing states' power to administer Medicaid funds may allow for savings through innovative, community-based solutions. Regardless of the overall effect of the DRA, patients and clinicians must expend energy to navigate decisions made by each state, which may even vary within a state.

Medicaid has become the default supplemental insurance for those who cannot afford Medicare Advantage or supplemental insurance. Unfortunately, even Medicaid is inadequately covering marginalized populations. Beneficiaries must apply separately for Medicare, Medicaid, and other supplemental assistance, which can be overwhelming, especially for people with pressing health concerns. Furthermore, this fragmented strategy increases administrative work for health care providers who must collect from the various payors and the third-party payors. Only 60% of people eligible for Medicare and Medicaid coverage received Medicaid benefits, with many spending 50% of their annual income on health care.[23] People with household incomes above the poverty level may not qualify for Medicaid,[24] but still find Medicare coverage insufficient.[25] These near-poverty beneficiaries spent up to 30% of their household income on health care and yet engaged in fewer outpatient visits and filled fewer medication prescriptions than those receiving Medicaid. For populations with a low socioeconomic status, the spotty coverage between Medicare, Medicaid, and supplemental insurance is expensive, inefficient, ineffective in delivering care, and unsustainable. The most recent assessment of Medicaid in 2019 demonstrated that for the 64 million people who were enrolled in Medicaid, annual expenditures were $386.5 billion with a projected growth rate of 4.4 to 5.3 resulting in more than $1 trillion annually by 2027.[26]

THE AFFORDABLE CARE ACT: 2010

The Affordable Care Act (ACA), developed during the Obama administration, consisting of Titles I through X was aimed at providing more affordable, quality, accessible and efficient health care to people of the United States.[27] A coordinated, bipartisan effort to provide a comprehensive, nationwide health policy had not been observed since the development of Medicare and Medicaid services. The ACA aimed to provide health care coverage for people through Medicare, Medicaid, subsidized Marketplace coverage, traditional health insurance, or some combination of these options. A particular focus was on the millions of uninsured and underinsured who did not qualify for Medicare and medicaid but could not afford marketplace health insurance coverage.[28] The ACA specifically addressed private insurers by creating the Marketplace, an opportunity to enroll the large population of uninsured and underinsured people. However, the ACA required that participating insurers cannot refuse coverage or charge more for coverage of those with preexisting conditions.[29] The ACA addressed individuals, particularly those who do not qualify for Medicaid or who cannot afford traditional private health insurance, by subsidizing the premiums of enrollees with incomes of 100% to 400% of the federal poverty level. Subsidies would ensure that no enrollee would have to pay more than 9.5% of their income in premiums. The ACA also offers cost-sharing reduction to individuals to defray the out-of-pocket costs, including deductibles, coinsurance, and copayments for eligible enrollees.[30] Individuals also faced an unprecedented penalty for not enrolling in health insurance.[31] Similarly, employers were subject to penalties paid to the Internal Revenue Service if they did not provide "affordable" health care insurance of "minimum value" to their full-time employees and dependents up to age 26.[32] If individuals can afford health insurance but choose not to buy it, they may be assessed a fee when filing federal taxes. The ACA addressed states' administration of Medicaid by allowing for federal funds to pay 90% of Medicaid expansion to people between 100% and 138% of the federal poverty level, thus narrowing the gap between those receiving Medicaid and those enrolling in subsidized insurance exchanges to private.

The implementation of the ACA's Medicaid expansion was reported by Sommers and colleagues,[33] who compared Kentucky's traditional Medicaid Expansion, Arkansas' use of Medicaid expansion funds to purchase private insurance (Private Option), and Texas' nonexpansion. Both forms of Medicaid expansion—traditional and Private Option—were associated with significantly increased access to primary care and specialty care, fewer incidences of skipped medications, reduced out-of-pocket spending, fewer emergency department visits, increased quality of care, and an increased number of people self-reporting excellent health. The implementation of the ACA has had variable effects on insurers.[34,35] The number of insurance companies participating in the Marketplace exchange increased from 2014 to 2015 upon the initial implementation of the ACA, but steadily declined from 2015 to 2018 likely because of poor financial performance. Interestingly, Medicaid-focused insurers had greater profit margins, perhaps because of their previous experience in managing these populations. However, the number of companies participating in the exchange market has increased over 2018 to 2021 and insurers remaining profitable, even during the coronavirus disease 2019 pandemic.[36]

What Does the ACA Do for Health Disparities?

The ACA has great potential to address disparities in health care. Before the ACA, many low-income populations reported lack of health insurance, financial barriers to medical care, and self-reported health; but rural populations faced an even greater disparity of health care options and professional shortages.[37] The ACA increased insurance coverage, health care access, and prescription drugs for 20 million low-income Americans.[38] Rural populations and minority populations demonstrated the greatest increases in insurance coverage, relationship with a personal physician, and obtaining medications.[33,39] The ACA also protects individuals from discrimination in procuring health insurance. The ACA specifically addressed equity in health care access and delivery to women; participating insurers cannot charge women more than men. People with preexisting conditions and disabilities are also protected from discrimination. By attracting private plans to the Marketplace exchange and through the expansion of Medicaid, the ACA assisted in developing health infrastructure and options in underserved urban and rural communities.[38] The ACA also established 6 offices of minority health to reside within 6 agencies of Health and Human Services namely Agency for Healthcare Research and

Quality (AHRQ), Center for Disease Control and Prevention (CDC), Centers for Medicare & Medicaid Services (CMS), Food and Drug Administration (FDA), Health Resources and Services Administration (HRSA), National Institute on Minority Health and Health Disparities (NIMHD) and Substance Abuse and Mental Health Services Administration (SAMHSA). Each of these agencies would have a common thread of accountability to the Office of Minority Health and thus health disparities.

Unfortunately, disparities in health care delivery persist. States that do not participate in Medicaid expansion have the highest poverty rates in the country.[40] Thus, several low-income people do not enjoy the insurance coverage benefits prescribed by the ACA. Even those with Medicaid and insurance procured on the ACA exchange have poorer access to health care providers than those with insurance procured privately or through employer-based programs.[41] Although the ACA has facilitated coverage for millions of Americans, a great proportion of those without health insurance before the implementation of the ACA remain uninsured.[42] In the most recent National Health Statistics Reports, 33 million persons remained uninsured.[43] Overall, 8% of Americans are uninsured including 15.9% of people living below the poverty level, 11.3% of people between 100% to 400% of the poverty level, and 3% of people above 400% of the poverty level.[44] Disparity of insurance by coverage by race and ethnicity persists, with a greater percentage of Black and African Americans (9.6%), Asians (6.2%), and Hispanics (16.7%) without coverage compared with White Americans (5.2%). Hispanic, Black, and African Americans continue to report worse access to routine care, specialty care and emergency care.[45] ACA has strategically sought to bring coverage to previously marginalized populations, but additional policies are needed to deliver health equity in the United States.

Durability of the Affordable Care Act

The ACA has faced several challenges, challenges that especially impact health care to people of lower income. In 2012, the US Supreme court decided in favor of the constitutionality of the ACA (*National Federation of Independent Business v. Sebelius*). However, this ruling gave states the choice whether or not to expand Medicaid to all individuals with incomes up to 138% of the federal poverty level.[46] In 2021, 12 states have yet to adopt the Medicaid expansion despite additional temporary incentive funds offered by the American Rescue Plan Act of 2021.[14] The House of Representatives posed an additional challenge to the ACA with a "repeal and replace" bill that passed in 2017. This proposed bill would give insurers the option to refuse or increase the cost of coverage based on preexisting conditions. Poorer populations be disproportionately harmed by this action because these populations likely to have comorbidities. Thus, resultant increased premiums and co-pays would have greater impact on those with low income. Among other financially based reductions, the proposed bill would eliminate subsidies for cost-sharing and reduction of health care expenses. The "repeal and replace" bill failed to gain support of the US Senate and perhaps reflected Americans' support of ACA. However, the Senate did move to eliminate the penalty to individuals who do not have health insurance. From 2017 to 2021, administrative actions undermined the ACA and potential enrollment of low-income Americans.[47] Reduction of enrollment periods for subsidized health insurance, reduction of funding for education and outreach regarding the ACA, the elimination of cost-sharing subsidies to decrease out-of-pocket health care expenses and short-term insurance plans resistant to restrictions of the ACA were implemented. It is unknown how these challenges to the ACA have impacted health and health disparities, but overall, the number of uninsured people has subtly increased from a low of 26.9 million in 2016 to 33.0 million in 2019.[43]

UNITED STATES EXECUTIVE BRANCH

Current and past Presidents of the United States have significantly influenced health and health disparities. This has occurred through the utilization of executive orders to enact a law passed by Congress or to exercise powers granted by the Constitution.[48] Since the passing of the Civil Rights Act in 1964, there have been multiple landmark executive orders that addressed health disparities. Executive Order 11,141 signed by Lyndon B. Johnson in 1964 declared a public policy against discriminating on the basis of age. This action was congruent with his campaign to develop both Medicare and Medicaid in 1965. With Executive Order 13,507, Barack Obama 2009 established a White House Office of Health Reform, within the Executive Office of the President, to improve access to health care, quality of care, and sustainability of the health care system as a whole. With Executive Order 13,544, Barack Obama in 2010 established the National Prevention, Health Promotion, and Public Health Council to address preventative health and wellness to the entirety of the United States population. With

Executive Order 13,941, issued by Donald Trump in 2020 aimed at improving sustainable health care for rural communities through the development of telehealth and communication. Executive Order 13,985 was the first executive order of Joseph Biden aimed at "Advancing Racial Equity and Support for Underserved Communities Through the Federal Government." This Executive Order established mechanisms and resources for assessment and intervention of inequities suffered by underserved communities. In Executive Order 13,995 by Joseph Biden 2021 allocates resources to combat racism with associated inequalities in health care and access and delivery exposed during the COVID-19 pandemic. In addition, President Biden has established the Office of Climate Change and Health Equity (OCCHE) to specifically address health equity.

Several government agencies have developed organizations to address health disparity. In 1953, President Eisenhower developed a Cabinet-level Department of Health, Education, and Welfare. In 1979, the Department of Education became its own entity and the Department of Health and Human Services, officially named in 1980, became the leading organization to address health disparities.[49] Margaret Heckler, Secretary of the Department of Health and Human Resources, led the Task Force on Black and Minority Health in 1985. The Task Force generated a report that showed shocking disparities in mortality and health disparities endured by all marginalized populations. They consolidated evidence which demonstrated that there were 6 disorders/entities which accounted for greater than 80% of mortality in ethnic and racial minorities, namely cancer, cardiovascular disease, chemical dependency, diabetes, homicides, and unintentional injuries. The report also stated recommendations that may aid in decreasing health disparities in these populations including outreach, education, improving access to care, promoting the quality of care, and integrating local, state, and federal agencies and support research in health disparities.[50] In 1979, Surgeon General Julius Richmond issued a landmark report titled "Healthy People: The Surgeon General's Report on Health Promotion and Disease Prevention," with an introductory letter from President Jimmy Carter. Then, in 1980, Office of Disease Prevention and Health Promotion (ODPHP) released Healthy People 1990 outlining measurable 10-year health objectives.[51] Every 10 years, new iterations of the Healthy People recommendations build on the last. The objectives of Healthy People 2000, 2010, 2020, and 2030 have evolved from identifying health disparities, to reducing health disparities, and eliminating health disparity as a priority. Now, numerous government agencies have invested in eliminating health disparities, including the Offices of Minority Health of Agency for Healthcare Research and Quality (AHRQ), the Centers for Disease Control and Prevention (CDC), the Centers for Medicare & Medicaid Services (CMS), the Food and Drug Administration (FDA), the Health Resources and Services Administration (HRSA), the National Institute on Minority Health and Health Disparities (NIMHD), the Substance Abuse and Mental Health Services Administration (SAMHSA), the Office of Minority Health & Health Disparities (OMHD), and the National Institutes of Health: Minority Health.

HEALTH LOBBYISTS

Health laws are not created in a vacuum. Health care lobbyists may represent patients, physicians, professional societies, health organizations, health industries, insurers, or any number of other stakeholders in the $3.8 trillion annual industry.[52] As new bills or issues are brought up at the state or federal levels, these groups use their influence to alter health policy in a way that benefits their respective interests. Their efforts can impact research priorities, the distribution of governmental or private funding, as well as the licensing, oversight, and distribution of health care products themselves. Possible outcomes impact the distribution of funds, products, licensing, oversight, and research priorities.

The 1995 Lobbying Disclosure Act required lobbyists to submit biannual reports describing activity and funds spent on lobbying. In health care lobbying expenditures totaled account for 15% of all federal lobbying, more than any other single industry.[52] Pharmaceutical and health product companies contribute an average of $233 million annually, consistently outspending any other lobbying interests.[53] Patients, especially those in marginalized groups, do not have the financing to compete in this process whatsoever. In 2001, lobbyists protecting interests of high-spending health insurance companies undermined a bipartisan Patient Bill of Rights 2001 that would have expanded Health Maintenance Organization coverage requirements and given employees the ability to sue employers for denial of claims. In 2019, the US Senate and the House proposed bills to protect patients from "surprise" billing. Surprise billing charges patients for out-of-network care, even when they have chosen an in-network physician/surgeon and in-network hospital. Surprise billing can come from out-of-network providers like anesthesiologists or surgical assistants, unbeknownst to the patient until after the procedure.

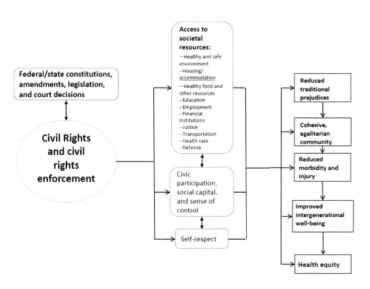

Fig. 2. Effects of civil rights laws on public health and health equity. (*From* Hahn RA, Truman BI, Williams DR. Civil rights as determinants of public health and racial and ethnic health equity: Health care, education, employment, and housing in the United States. SSM Popul Health. 2018;4:17-24.)

Unfortunately, private equity firms and physician groups have leveraged lobbyists in opposition to these bills with no matching advocacy from patients. Fortunately, in 2021 HHS published an interim final rule aimed at banning the practice of surprise billing, but lobbying interest and specialty groups have vowed to oppose the rule.

DISCUSSION

Health policy encompasses laws, implementation. and enforcement. The US Legislative, Judicial, and Executive Branches have recognized and endeavored to address health disparities. However, eliminating health disparity requires that we acknowledge injustice and structural discrimination,[54] not only in health policy but other social determinants including housing, employment, transportation, education, security, economy and environment. Civil right laws directly impact public health, health equity and individual's health.[55] **(Fig. 2)** Health disparities are not simply variable health outcomes, but "systematic, plausibly avoidable health differences. . . associated with discrimination or marginalization." Through acknowledging core human rights of equality and health, we have the potential to realize optimal health status for each person. Although some significant strides have been made through the last 50 year to improve healthcare equity, much still remains to be done. A recent article investigated changes within racial and ethnic subgroups over two decades with regard to self-reported personal health status as well as healthcare access and affordability. The authors found that there has been some moderate improvement in health disparities within racial and ethnic subgroups, significant inequities persist despite the past 5 decades, legislative and regulatory activity. The proposed Health Equity and Accountability Act of 2020 will challenge the ideological and practical limits of health equity. This bill includes provisions for noncitizens. The future of the ACA and discussion surrounding the proposed Medicare for All Act of 2021 will continue to test the value our nation places on health and health equity.

Although the challenge of health equity seems overwhelming, the Veterans Health Administration (VHA) has prioritized health equity and committed research, detection, understanding determinants, reduction and elimination of health disparities. In a recent review of more than 25 studies, the VHA, has reduced many mortality disparities including similar or lower mortality for Black veterans compared with White veterans.[56] While disparity in certain clinical areas and with other marginalized groups persist, hopefully we can learn from the VHA experience to make concrete, durable and meaningful progress in at least access to health care.

In thoracic surgery, health disparities not only impact our patients, but also our workforce, health systems, reimbursement, and our research funding. It is imperative that we develop shared values of equality and health. From here we can build infrastructure to advance health equity as individuals or as part of institutions, professional societies or political action committees. At this time, silence and inaction will perpetuate health disparities.

CLINICS CARE POINTS

- The history of health care policy demonstrates structural inequities that contribute to health disparities in the United States.
- A fundamental knowledge of Medicare, Medicaid, and the ACA is necessary to understand reimbursement for thoracic surgical services and practice.
- Navigating the complex system of insurance is difficult, but even more so for patients with low health literacy, low income, low education, low English proficiency, and low trust.
- Silence and inaction will perpetuate health disparities. We as thoracic surgeons can mitigate health disparities through our patient care, education, research, innovation, and health policy advocacy.

DISCLOSURE

This work was partially supported by TUFCCC/HC Regional Comprehensive Cancer Health Disparity Partnership, Award Number U54 CA221704(5) (Contact PIs: Grace X. Ma, PhD and Olorunseun O. Ogunwobi, MD, PhD) from the National Cancer Institute of National Institutes of Health (NCI/NIH) and The American Cancer Society – Pfizer Health Disparities Grant. The content is solely the responsibility of the authors and does not necessarily represent the official views of the funding agencies.

REFERENCES

1. Available at: https://www.cms.gov/Research-Statistics-Data-and-Systems/Statistics-Trends-and-Reports/NationalHealthExpendData/NHE-Fact-Sheet. Accessed September 15, 2021.
2. McGowan a, Lee MM, Meneses CM, et al. Civil rights laws as tools to advance health in the twenty-first century. Annu Rev Public Health 2016; 37:185–204.
3. Available at: https://pnhp.org/news/getting-martin-luther-kings-words-right/. Accessed September 15, 2021.
4. Reynolds PP. Hospitals and civil rights, 1945-1963: the case of simkins v Moses H. Cone Memorial Hospital. Ann Intern Med 1997;126:898–906.
5. The Civil Rights Act of 1964: eleven titles at a glance. Available at: https://crsreports.congress.gov. Accessed September 15, 2021.
6. DiPolito SA. Olmstead v. l.c. deinstitutionalization and community integration: an awakening of the nation's conscience. Mercer L Rev 2007;58(4): 1381–410.
7. Perone AK. Health implications of the supreme court's Obergefell vs. Hodges Marriage Equality Decision. LGBT health 2015;2(3):196–9.
8. Available at: https://www.hhs.gov/civil-rights/for-providers/laws-regulations-guidance/laws/index.html.
9. Smith DB. Racial and ethnic health disparities and the unfinished civil rights agenda. Health Aff (Millwood) 2005;24(2):317–24.
10. Origins of the Medicare Kidney disease entitlement: the social security amendments of 1972. In: Institute of Medicine (US) Committee to Study Decision Making, Hanna KE, editors. Biomedical politics. Washington (DC): National Academies Press (US); 1991. Available at: https://www.ncbi.nlm.nih.gov/books/NBK234191/.
11. Available at: https://www.ssa.gov/policy/docs/ssb/v50n12/v50n12p13.pdf. Accessed September 15, 2021.
12. Schoen C, Buttorff C, Andersen M, et al. Policy options to expand Medicare's low-income provisions to improve access and affordability. Health Aff (Millwood) 2015;34(12):2086–94.
13. McGuire TG, Newhouse JP, Sinaiko AD. An economic history of Medicare part C [published correction appears in Milbank Q. 2013 Mar;91(1):210. Milbank Q 2011;89(2):289–332.
14. Available at: https://www.kff.org/medicare/issue-brief/medicare-advantage-in-2021-enrollment-update-and-key-trends/.
15. Brunt CS. Supplemental insurance and racial health disparities under Medicare part B. Health Serv Res 2017;52(6):2197–218.
16. Eichner J, Vladeck BC. Medicare as a catalyst for reducing health disparities. Health Aff (Millwood) 2005;24(2):365–75.
17. Day CL. Older Americans' attitudes toward the Medicare catastrophic coverage act of 1988. J Polit 1993;55(1):167–77.
18. Tailor TD, Tong BC, Gao J, et al. Utilization of Lung Cancer Screening in the Medicare Fee-for-Service Population. Chest 2020;158(5):2200–10.
19. Available at: https://www.kff.org/medicaid/poll-finding/medicare-and-medicaid-at-50/. Accessed September 15, 2021.
20. Rosenbaum S, Wise PH. Crossing the Medicaid-private insurance divide: the case of EPSDT. Health Aff (Millwood) 2007;26(2):382–93.
21. Soman L, Smith K, Duenas J. The Federal Deficit Reduction Act and its impact on children. J Pediatr Nurs 2008;23(5):386–92.
22. Available at: https://aspe.hhs.gov/topics/poverty-economic-mobility/poverty-guidelines/prior-hhs-poverty-guidelines-federal-register-references/

2021-poverty-guidelines. Accessed September 15, 2021.

23. Gross DJ, Alecxih L, Gibson MJ, et al. Out-of-pocket health spending by poor and near-poor elderly Medicare beneficiaries. Health Serv Res 1999;34(1 Pt 2):241–54.

24. Schoen C, Davis K, Buttorff C, et al. Modernizing Medicare's benefit design and low-income subsidies to ensure access and affordability. Issue Brief (Commonw Fund) 2015;21:1–13.

25. Roberts ET, Glynn A, Cornelio N, et al. Medicaid Coverage 'Cliff' Increases Expenses And Decreases Care For Near-Poor Medicare Beneficiaries. Health Aff (Millwood) 2021;40(4):552–61.

26. Available at: https://www.cms.gov/newsroom/factsheets/medicaid-facts-and-figures. Accessed September 15, 2021.

27. Obamacare Act: a summary of its 10 Titles. Available at: https://www.thebalance.com/obamacare-bill-3306057. Accessed September 15, 2021.

28. Available at: https://aspe.hhs.gov/sites/default/files/private/pdf/265041/trends-in-the-us-uninsured.pdf. Accessed September 15, 2021.

29. Available at: https://www.healthcare.gov/coverage/pre-existing-conditions/. Accessed September 15, 2021

30. Available at: https://www.healthcare.gov/glossary/com. Accessed September 15, 2021.

31. Available at: https://www.healthcare.gov/fees/fee-for-not-being-covered/. Accessed September 15, 2021.

32. Available at: https://www.irs.gov/affordable-care-act/employers/employer-shared-responsibility-provisions. Accessed September 15, 2021.

33. Sommers BD, Blendon RJ, Orav EJ, et al. Changes in utilization and health among low-income adults after Medicaid expansion or expanded private insurance. JAMA Intern Med 2016;176(10):1501–9.

34. Hall MA, McCue MJ. How Has the Affordable Care Act affected health insurers' financial performance? Issue Brief (Commonw Fund) 2016;18:1–14.

35. McCue M, Hall MA, Palazzolo J. Key drivers of financial performance of insurers in the Affordable Care Act market exchange. Health Serv Manage Res 2020.

36. Available at: https://www.kff.org/private-insurance/issue-brief/insurer-participation-on-the-aca-marketplaces-2014-2021/.

37. Andrulis DP, Siddiqui NJ, Purtle JP, et al. Patient protection and affordable care Act of 2010: advancing health equity for racially and ethnically diverse populations. Washington, DC: Joint Center for Political and Economic Studies; 2010.

38. Hasnain-Wynia R, Beal AC. The path to equitable health care. Health Serv Res 2012;47(4):1411–7.

39. Benitez JA, Seiber EE. US health care reform and rural America: results from the ACA's Medicaid expansions. J Rural Health 2018;34(2):213–22.

40. Adepoju OE, Preston MA, Gonzales G. Health care disparities in the post-affordable care act era. Am J Public Health (1971) 2015;105(Suppl 5):S665–7.

41. Alcalá HE, Roby DH, Grande DT, et al. Insurance type and access to health care providers and appointments under the affordable care act. Med Care 2018;56(2):186–92.

42. Gaffney A, McCormick D. The Affordable Care Act: implications for health-care equity. Lancet 2017;389(10077):1442–52.

43. Available at: https://www.cdc.gov/nchs/data/nhsr/nhsr159-508.pdf. Accessed September 15, 2021.

44. Available at: http://www.census.gov/content/dam/Census/library/publications/2020/demo/p60-271.pdf. Accessed September 15, 2021

45. Available at: https://www.ahrq.gov/sites/default/files/wysiwyg/research/findings/nhqrdr/2019qdr.pdf. Accessed September 15, 2021.

46. Levitt L. The Affordable Care Act's enduring resilience. J Health Polit Policy Law 2020;45(4):609–16.

47. Available at: https://www.kff.org/policy-watch/what-we-do-and-dont-know-about-recent-trends-in-health-insurance-coverage-in-the-us/. Accessed September 15, 2021.

48. Available at: https://www.phe.gov/s3/law/Pages/ExecOrders.aspx. Accessed September 15, 2021.

49. Available at: https://www.hhs.gov/about/historical-highlights/index.html.

50. Report of the Secretary's Task Force on Black and Minority Health. Available at: https://collections.nlm.nih.gov/catalog/nlm:nlmuid-8602912-mvset. Accessed September 15, 2021.

51. Available at: https://health.gov/our-work/national-health-initiatives/healthy-people/about-healthy-people/history-healthy-people. Accessed September 15, 2021.

52. Landers SH, Sehgal AR. Health care lobbying in the United States. Am J Med 2004;116(7):474–7.

53. Wouters OJ. Lobbying expenditures and campaign contributions by the pharmaceutical and health product industry in the United States, 1999-2018. JAMA Intern Med 2020;180(5):688–97.

54. Braveman PA, Kumanyika S, Fielding J, et al. Health disparities and health equity: the issue is justice. Am J Public Health 2011;101(Suppl 1):S149–55.

55. Hahn RA, Truman BI, Williams DR. Civil rights as determinants of public health and racial and ethnic health equity: health care, education, employment, and housing in the United States. SSM Popul Health 2018;4:17–24.

56. Peterson K, Anderson J, Boundy E, et al. Mortality disparities in racial/ethnic minority groups in the veterans health administration: an evidence review and map. Am J Public Health 2018;108(3):e1–11.

Disparities in Health Care Delivery Systems

Muhammad Farhan Nadeem, MD[a], Larry R. Kaiser, MD[b,c],*

KEYWORDS

- Health care disparities • Health care delivery • Health care utilization • Racial disparities
- COVID-19 • Affordable care act • Social determinants of health

KEY POINTS

- Racial disparities have been increasing in health care delivery systems and stem from increasing socioeconomic inequality.
- Despite efforts to improve primary care, for example, Affordable Care Act, the emergency room continues to be the primary means to attain medical care for underrepresented minority populations.
- COVID-19 pandemic threatens to increase the disparity gap, demanding innovative approaches to deliver equitable health services.

Health care in the United States is unique than other developed countries. Most other countries have health care systems controlled and provided by the government that provides health care for all. This results in a system whereby health care is a right and citizens are entitled to it. However, in the United States, the system is fragmented, has multiple components, and complexities that make access difficult for many and unfortunately result in almost 15% of the population without coverage. This leads to multiple inequalities in health care delivery which we review in this paper.

OPTIMAL HEALTH CARE DELIVERY SYSTEM CHARACTERISTICS

Optimal health care, if it were to truly exist, would be defined as access for all and timely delivery of affordable personal health services that achieve the best health outcomes. Ideally, the system would be designed to maintain wellness as well as treat the sick and infirmed. The above definition is an oversimplification and is packed with cues of social injustice. To understand the disparities inherent in health care delivery systems, it is mandatory to review an ideal health care delivery system and the phases for which the care is delivered.

PHASES OF HEALTH CARE DELIVERY AND ASSOCIATED INEQUALITIES
Timely Access

Accessibility to health care, in addition to the ability to obtain physical access to a physician or hospital, pertains to the ability to enter the system in a timely fashion.

Timeliness is probably the most important factor that affects accessibility as indicated by patient satisfaction surveys. Not only patient satisfaction but prolonged emergency room wait times can lead to increased mortality.[1–3] Multiple studies have shown that black patients wait significantly longer for emergency room care than nonblack patients. On average, black patients experienced significantly longer mean emergency room wait times than white patients (69.2 vs 53.3 minutes; $P<.001$).[4] However, it was also noted that the size of disparity in wait times became more pronounced as the severity of illness decreased. The emergency room is not the ideal place for individuals to receive primary care, yet it often is the most

a Temple University Hospital, 3401 N Broad Street, Philadelphia, PA 19140, USA; b Alvarez & Marsal, 600 Madison Avenue, 8th Floor, New York, NY 10022, USA; c University of Pennsylvania Perelman School of Medicine
* Corresponding author. Alvarez & Marsal, 600 Madison Avenue, 8th Floor, New York, NY 10022.
E-mail address: lkaiser@alvarezandmarsal.com

Thorac Surg Clin 32 (2022) 13–21
https://doi.org/10.1016/j.thorsurg.2021.09.005
1547-4127/22/© 2021 Elsevier Inc. All rights reserved.

readily available and accessible venue for the underserved. Multiple studies have shown that access to primary care is associated with positive health outcomes. The National Academy of Medicine defines primary care as "the provision of integrated, accessible health care services by a clinician who is accountable for addressing most of the personal health care needs, developing a sustained partnership with patients, and practicing in the context of family and community. Certainly, this type of wraparound care provides significant advantages over episodic care in a busy emergency department whereby the continuity of care is challenging, at best. Primary care providers include individuals from internal medicine, family medicine, pediatrics, nurse practitioners (NPs), physician assistants (PAs), and obstetrics and gynecology. Some obstacles to accessing primary care include the lack of insurance, language barriers, disabilities, inability to take time off work, and a shortage of primary care providers located within certain populations.

Insurance Coverage

There is enormous variation between racial groups when it comes to insurance coverage and its effects on access to health care. African American and Hispanic populations in the United States are more likely to be uninsured throughout adulthood than non-Hispanic or white individuals.[5] In addition to simply being able to obtain health insurance, the ability to maintain insurance is also of utmost importance as interruptions to one's care is more likely to occur with frequent insurance loss and subsequent regain. Also, National surveys have shown that the best experiences are reported by patients who are able to and have the means to obtain private insurance.[5]

Geographic Availability of Services

Geographic accessibility of health care services, whereby access to care is reasonably nearby, has been associated with favorable health outcomes. Community health centers (CHCs) are vital in the provision of primary care for the poor and underserved. They serve 25 million patients at more than 11,000 CHC sites. Most of the patients who use CHC's for their health care are disproportionately poor and underserved with about 92% having incomes less than 200% of the federal poverty level, 62% are minorities, and 73% have Medicaid or are uninsured.[6]

The monitoring of CHCs is conducted by the Health Resources and Services Administration (HRSA). The Affordable Care Act (ACA) of 2010 allocated 9.5 billion dollars between 2011 and 2015 to new sites and service expansion. HRSA mandates that CHCs should be established in medically underserved areas. The Index of Medical Underservice (IMU) is used to select areas with IMU less than 63 that would then qualify as a medically underserved area. This index is determined by the proportion of the population in poverty, the primary care physician to population ratio, the proportion of the area population more than 65, and the infant mortality rate. Though the system is objective, there are multiple problems associated with the distribution of these centers. The IMU threshold of 63 was defined in the 1970s and has not been updated since that time and this designation does not account for different levels of medical under service. In addition, the IMU does not account for several significant social determinants, beyond poverty level and age, well known to be associated with disparities.[7]

Provision of Services

In addition to the disparities in access, insurance coverage, and geographic availability for services, the provision of quality health care also varies by ethnic groups. How a patient experiences care is one element of overall quality but may be a limiting factor is a patient actually seeking care if the experience has been poor. The Consumer Assessment of Health care Providers and Systems (CAHPSs) is a widely used tool to assess a patient's care experience.

Asian Americans with limited English proficiency (LEP) have been reported to have lower rates of satisfactory patient experience though blacks and Hispanics often report a health care experience comparable to non-Hispanic whites.[8] The role of unconscious bias must also be considered whenever one considers the patient experience. Unfortunately, this type of bias exists among many providers and as well as institutions but recognizing it has made some inroads into reducing the effect.

Preventive care should be a major part of primary care with the ultimate outcome being the maintenance of wellness, which if used effectively could result in major cost savings within the health care system. Any barrier to the provision of quality primary care results in a lapse of preventive medicine. For example, cancer screening is lower in blacks, Hispanics, American Indians, and some Asian groups. Generally, rural residents have lower rates of being screened for various cancers; however, paradoxically African American women have higher rates of cancer screening than white women.[9] Also with Medicaid being run by each individual state, there remain significant differences in eligibility depending on the location. These differences result in some of the biggest gaps in cancer screening in addition to a similar trend in adult immunization.

Similarly, the care of common chronic diseases varies in different population groups with minority patients having poorer control of blood pressure, blood sugar, cholesterol, and HIV. Social determinants such as food and housing insecurity as well as transportation challenges all play into this disparity. Access challenges as well as some residual distrust of the health system based on historical perspectives also contribute to poorer control of these common conditions. Can some of these disparities be addressed by greater access with the rise of "retail medicine," specifically the development of urgent care centers and health care delivery at the local CVS or Rite Aid? Perhaps, but once again the lack of insurance is a barrier for many and often the urgent care centers demand cash upfront, whether one has insurance or not.

Even for inpatient admissions, minority populations fair worse with African Americans having higher rates of readmission following hospitalization for potentially avoidable causes such as asthma, diabetes, heart failure, and postsurgical complications.[10] There is also significant evidence indicating that minority populations use behavioral health services, including substance use disorder treatment, less often than non-Hispanic white patients, thought access to these services remains challenging for multiple populations due to a lack of supply to meet the increasing demand.

HEALTH CARE DELIVERY AFTER THE AFFORDABLE CARE ACT

The ACA was signed by President Barack Obama on March 23, 2010. The ACA's major provisions, which were fully accessible in 2014, resulted in decreasing by almost 50% in the number of uninsured individuals by 2016 with an estimated 20 to 24 million additional people gaining insurance. It also included a variety of reforms intended to reduce the growth in health care costs while improving the quality.[11]

This increased coverage resulted both from the expansion of Medicaid eligibility and the creation of state and federal insurance exchanges, which allowed for individuals to purchase a plan that met their needs often accompanied by a subsidy provided by the federal government that increased the affordability of the coverage. Despite the availability of several options offered through the exchanges, if one does not qualify for a subsidy the

options available may still be too expensive. Part of the reason for this was the requirement that all plans offered through the exchanges had to offer certain prescribed basic coverage, much of which many individuals do not need. In addition, in certain markets, there may only be one insurer offering plans, which may result in increased cost as there is no competition. Medicare, Medicaid, and the employer market retained their existing structures whereas individual markets underwent significant changes. No longer could individuals be denied coverage based on preexisting illness, and insurers could not penalize those with such illnesses by charging more. Also, mandated was insurance for children who did not have coverage via their families through the Children's Health Insurance Program (CHIP). Insurance companies were forbidden from dropping policyholders when they became ill. There was a special emphasis placed on preventive medicine and primary care as well with the major aim to reduce cost while maintaining and ideally improving quality. Additional provisions included.

- A 10% increase in Medicare primary care reimbursement rates, 2011 to 2016 ($3.5 Billion)
- Medicaid reimbursement for primary care increased to at least Medicare levels, 2013 to 14 ($8.3 Billion)
- Scholarships, loan repayment, and training demonstration programs to invest in primary care providers and community providers.
- Patient-centered medical homes, primary care sites that provided the availability of appointments after regular office hours in addition to the team approach to medical care involving not just the physician but NPs, dieticians, pharmacists, and social workers. The intent was to create something greater than taking care of people when they got sick but truly addressing wellness and continued care especially of chronic disease.

ROOT CAUSE OF HEALTH DISPARITIES: UNEQUAL DISTRIBUTION OF RESOURCES

With the provisions mandated by the ACA, insurance exchanges and Medicaid expansion were able to provide health coverage for a significant proportion of the previously uninsured population. However, the structural barriers remained untouched that prevented these changes to percolate to the extremely poor. These structural barriers include income and racial health inequalities, and we will discuss them later in detail.

COVERAGE GAP: IMPLICATIONS OF NOT ALL STATES ADOPTING MEDICAID EXPANSION

Under the ACA funding of Medicaid was significantly expanded. In addition to enhanced funding, Medicaid eligibility was expanded to include all US citizens and qualified noncitizens up to age 64 with incomes up to 138% (133% plus a 5% income disregard) of the federal poverty level. This included adults without dependent children. However, the Supreme Court of the United States ruled in the National Federation of Independent Business versus Sebelius[12] that states did not have to agree to this expansion to continue to receive previously established levels of Medicaid funding.

Currently, 10 states, Florida, Georgia, Kansas, Mississippi, North Carolina, South Carolina, South Dakota, Texas, Wisconsin, and Wyoming, have not yet adopted Medicaid expansions. Missouri and Oklahoma have adopted but not yet implemented the expansion.

Medicaid expansion has resulted in gains in coverage, improvements in access, financial security, and some measures of health status/outcomes as well as economic benefits for states and providers. In addition, Medicaid expansion states have shown a decrease in overall mortality. With these gains in mind, it is worth exploring the implications for the coverage gap. Adults who fall into the coverage gap have incomes above their state's eligibility for Medicaid but below poverty, the minimum income eligibility for tax credits through the ACA marketplace. Medicaid eligibility for adults in nonexpansion states is quite limited, with the median income limit of just 41% of the federal poverty level, or an annual income of $8905 for a family of 3 in 2020. In nearly all states, not expanding childless adults remain ineligible. In contrast, in states that have adopted Medicaid expansion, eligibility is extended to nearly all low-income individuals with incomes at or less than 138% of poverty ($17,609 for an individual in 2020).[13]

Nationally, more than 2 million uninsured adults fell into the coverage gap that resulted from state decisions not to expand Medicaid, meaning their income was above Medicaid eligibility but below the lower limit for Marketplace premium tax credits. Most people who fell within the coverage Gap, about 77%, are adults without dependent children, and most of these people are in the southern United States. Most of these states have large populations of people of color, and the decision not to expand their programs disproportionately affects people of color, particularly black Americans.

RETAIL CLINICS IN THE UNITED STATES

The rise of "retail medicine" in the form of the urgent care center and walk-in clinics has made health care significantly more accessible and convenient at least for a portion of the population. Many of these facilities are in supermarkets, pharmacies, and retail stores and usually treat uncomplicated minor illnesses. These are usually staffed by NPs and PAs whereas some are staffed by physicians.

As of 2015, more than 2000 retail clinics were available in the United States and at that time had provided 35 million patient visits. They have the capacity to provide care through over 10 million patient visits per year. One of the major reasons for the success of retail medicine has been ease of access at a convenient location with the flexibility of appointment (usually walk-ins) and lower costs (a wellness visit at Walmart costs $59 and cholesterol screening at CVS is $59 to $69). In addition to the presence of clinics in some Walmart stores, the company has now opened 3 free-standing health and wellness facilities that offer a full range of services including dental and optical. Prices are posted online, and patients can see exactly what a visit will cost in advance. It has been shown that the quality of primary care provided at these retail clinics is comparable, if not superior to the care offered in doctor's office and emergency department settings.[14]

One of the indicators of expanding stakes of retail clinics in health care is the presence of partnerships between the hospitals, clinics, and health systems. More than 100 such partnerships are present throughout the county, and the number is steadily growing.

CVS has created HealthHUB in several of their stores around the country whereby primary care visits are offered, and the intent is to manage chronic illness as well as minor medical problems. CVS, following the merger with Aetna, is now the "front door" for Aetna beneficiaries and it was recently announced that behavioral health services will be offered in some locations. CVS is in the process of reconfiguring several of its stores to accommodate these HealthHUBs. In 2006, CVS acquired Minute Clinic, which put them into the retail health business and now they have more than, is 1100 locations in 33 states and the District of Columbia.

Retail clinics are interested in both complementing and potentially competing with primary care physicians but with the added convenience of easier access. Most of the population of the United States is within 5 miles of a CVS store. For the uninsured retail, clinics present a challenge in that they require cash for a visit. Unlike emergency rooms that do not require cash before being seen, both urgent care centers and retail outlets demand cash payment and usually do not accept those with Medicaid further contributing to the disparity in health care delivery. Yes, they do offer convenience but seemingly not for all. Interestingly, the American Academy of Pediatrics in 2014 came out with a recommendation against the use of retail clinics. This was subsequently revised in another statement from AAP in 2017 stating, "The Academy recommends that physicians coordinate with urgent care and retail-based clinics, to ensure high-quality services outside the medical home."

With the COVID-19 pandemic, retail clinics played a significant role in providing drive-thru/on-site testing at a multitude of locations though nothing is perfect and delays in receiving results, lost specimens, and poor customer service have been reported.

INCREASED TRANSPARENCY AFTER THE ACA AND CONSUMER PROTECTION

The ACA made it mandatory for insurance companies to use plain language in describing benefits and coverage. Before the ACA, financial and medical jargon could lead to significant miscommunication between the insurance provider and the consumer as to what coverage to expect after purchasing insurance and what insurance options existed. A short, easy-to-understand Summary of Benefits and Coverage (or SBC) was standardized as a comparison tool for the general public. A glossary of terms commonly used in health insurance coverage such as "deductible" and "copayment" was also made mandatory.

In addition to increased transparency requirements for insurance companies, hospital price transparency is another feature of the ACA. Hospitals now are required to make their prices available online by publishing their "Chargemasters" or list prices for all services provided. This resulted in complicated lists of thousands of goods and services on thousands of individual websites, which even for sophisticated consumers, are difficult to interpret.

Even with chargemaster prices listed rice comparison is hard if not impossible. As the total cost for needed treatments is hard to predict, especially for emergency services and for complex medical problems, all prediction tools fall short of giving an accurate estimate and thus an accurate comparison. In addition, costs reflected on list-price data do not reflect the prices that are relevant for patients. For example, in a knee replacement surgery, the costs of the inventory used might be different for different patients based on insurance negotiated rates, deductibles, coinsurance, and copayments.

And finally, patients usually do not have the adequate knowledge required to make a fair cost comparison as they do not know the quality of services provided to them. It is also impossible for patients to make judgments regarding quality and must rely on their primary care physician or whoever referred them.

OUT-OF-NETWORK AND SURPRISE BILLING

Surprise bills often arise in emergencies whereby patients have little control over care received when they present to an emergency room and are seen by a variety of consultants. They also arise in nonemergencies when patients present to locations or practitioners who do not participate in the network in which they are enrolled. Most commonly patients are completely unaware they are being seen by someone out of network as that information usually is not disclosed at the time of treatment. Thus, the surprise, and not a pleasant one, arrives when the patient receives a bill, usually a large one for which they were unprepared.

In one survey, 66% of the adults said that they worried about unexpected medical bills more than any other health care or household expense.[15] Among patients with private insurance, surprise billing affects 1 in 5 emergency claims and 1 in 6 in-network hospitalizations. Some plans might outwardly deny the out-of-network care or they might pay a portion of the bill, but the balance falls to the patient to pay. This balance can easily approach thousands of dollars. For those covered by Medicare and Medicaid, surprise billing is not an issue.

In the closing days of 2020, Congress signed the No Surprise Act, which when it goes into effect in 2022, mandates private health plans to cover surprise medical bills for emergency services as well as out-of-network provider charges at an in-network facility. Also, the Act prohibits balance billing for surprise bills beyond the applicable in-network cost-sharing amount.[15]

BARRIERS TO DELIVERY
Health Literacy

The definition of health literacy was updated in August 2020 with the release of Healthy People 2030 that divides it into 2 components. Personal health literacy is the degree to which individuals can find, understand, and use information and services to inform health-related decisions and actions for themselves and others. Organizational health literacy is the degree to which organizations equitably enable individuals to find, understand, and use information and services to inform health-related decisions and actions for themselves and others. Health literacy has been found to be associated with several other drivers of health disparities that include, but are not limited to, socioeconomic status, education, and income. Studies have shown that non-Whites have limited health literacy than Whites.[16,17] It has also been demonstrated that health literacy mediated or effectively reduced the effect of race/ethnicity and education on self-reported general health, which includes both physical and mental health. Another study found that LEP was a more important predictor than health literacy in explaining self-reported health status in Hispanics, Vietnamese, Whites, and other races.[18,19]

High Cost of Care

In a 2019 survey, 1 in every 10 Americans reported cost to be a barrier to access health care and they either did not receive or delayed receiving medical care because of costs. Of these Americans, 15.1% were Hispanics, 13% non-Hispanic Blacks, 9.3% non-Hispanic Whites, and 4.8% were Asians. Paradoxically adults in poorer health, according to this survey, were twice as likely to delay care or go without care due to high costs.[20]

Inadequate or No Insurance

Not surprisingly, the 2019 survey also confirmed that uninsured adults delaying or going without care due to cost is higher than insured adults. Of uninsured adults, 37% said that they delayed or went without health care because of cost than 7% of insured adults. The survey also revealed that the share of uninsured delaying or going without care increased by 3% points between 2016 and 2018, whereas the share of insured individuals changed by less than 1% over the same time period.[21] Uninsured individuals were also noted to be three times more likely to use urgent care or an emergency room as their routine and preferred site of care.

Lack of Availability of Services

Limited availability of health care resources is another barrier that may reduce access to health services and increase the risk for poor health outcomes. This is especially true in areas whereby poor people live in addition to rural areas of the country.

Lack of Cultural Competency

The ability to relate and empathize with individuals from different cultures and origins is an important part of a patient's health care experience and has been correlated with improved health care outcomes. It has been estimated that fully one-half of the US population will be comprised of minorities by 2050.[22] This further underscores the rationale for health care providers to understand and recognize the presence of diverse cultures and the importance of catering to the needs of individual cultures.

Promoting diversity and inclusivity is an important component of improving the cultural competence of the system. Providing educational materials and signage in different languages recognizing food preferences and restrictions of patients based on religious or ethnic reasons and promoting a culture of inclusion are some of the ways to make a system culturally sensitive.

Unconscious (Implicit) Bias

An Institute of Medicine report concluded that unrecognized bias against members of a social group whether based on race or ethnicity can adversely affect the quality of care offered to those individuals.[23] It is critically important that one recognizes the existence of unconscious bias despite being unaware of it and education directed specifically toward this recognition has been shown to be of great use. The implicit association test (IAT), which is a computerized, timed dual categorization test, measures implicit preferences by bypassing conscious control.[24] The IAT has consistently demonstrated a pro-white bias in most of the test-takers. Compared with non-black physicians, black physicians, not surprisingly, demonstrated less pro-white bias. The correlation between implicit bias and poor health care provision has been established in a study showing high pro-white IAT results and black patients' perception of poor-quality care and communication.[25]

Lack of Trust in Health Care Systems Especially Larger Systems

National surveys have shown that there is an abundance of distrust on the part of many regarding the health care system in the United States. This distrust is higher among uninsured individuals and those between 31 and 60 years of age. Non-Hispanic black responders were more likely than non-Hispanic white responders to be concerned about personal privacy and the potential for harmful" experimentation" in larger hospitals. Distrust of the health care system is associated with poorer self-reported health even after adjusting for age, sex, education, income, and insurance coverage.[26]

Lack of Transportation or Child Care

A large secondary analysis of National Health interview survey data, medical expenditure panel survey data, and Bureau of Transportation statistics data estimated that 3.6 million people are unable to access medical care due to issues dealing with transportation. These individuals were more likely to be older, poorer, less educated, female, and from ethnic minority groups. Also, individuals with the highest burden of disease tend to have the highest burden of transportation barriers. In another analysis, American Indian/Alaskan Natives were more likely to delay care due to transportation problems.

In a similar study, African Americans had greater issues relating to travel than Whites, defined as greater than 30 mins to access care, even after controlling for socioeconomic status.[27]

Transportation barriers often result in missed clinic appointments, rescheduled medical appointments, timely access to pharmacy, and thus medications and medication refills and worse clinical outcomes.

COVID-19 RESPONSE EXPOSING RACIAL DISPARITIES

It has now been conclusively demonstrated that preexisting chronic conditions including obesity, diabetes, hypertension, cardiovascular disease, cigarette smoking, and chronic obstructive pulmonary disease are significant risk factors for the hospitalization of COVID-19 patients. It has been estimated that 45.4% of US adults are at increased risk for complications from COVID-19. In the United States, it has been established that minority populations have much higher COVID-19 mortality with the reasons likely to be multifactorial. For example, in Chicago, African Americans comprise 30% of the population, yet they accounted for 50% of COVID-19 patients and 70% of COVID-19 deaths, mostly concentrated in a small number of vulnerable communities.

The high COVID-19 incidence and morbidity and mortality rate in a minority population can be at least partly explained by a higher prevalence of hypertension and cardiovascular disease in African American populations. Hispanic and African American communities have the highest rates of poor outpatient diabetic control and a higher incidence of diabetes-related complications and hospital admissions. Whether these chronic conditions might be related to poor access to basic preventive medical care remains unknown but there is no question of the disparity between this population and the Caucasian population.

INNOVATIVE MODELS OF PRIMARY CARE DELIVERY AND THEIR ROLE IN COVID-19 AND TELEHEALTH

Primary care practices have been under immense financial pressure, especially since the outbreak of the COVID-19 pandemic. Fewer than 10% of primary care practices have stabilized operations amid the pandemic. The struggling primary care practices have suffered from a lack of funding despite the CARES Act. One estimate indicates that just 5 to 7% of health care funding is provided to outpatient primary care in the United States. In comparison, primary care accounts for an average of 14% of the total health care spending across first-world European countries. Our predominant fee-for-service (FFS) payment model is fundamentally misaligned with the nature of continuous, comprehensive, and coordinated primary care.

In the realm of primary care, newer startups that are based on value-based payment models have become much more prevalent. These startups are accountable for the total cost, quality, and experience of care and are paid on a per member per month basis that presents both an upside and downside risk. They offer integrated, team-based care in a patient-centered manner and get rewarded for establishing systems that function to maintain health while reducing costs primarily by avoiding hospital admissions and emergency room visits.

Some examples of these innovative approaches to care for at-risk populations include:

City Block: (Medicaid)
   This Alphabet spinoff offers primary care, behavioral health, substance use disorder treatment, and virtual care services for underserved communities; it also developed a virtual pregnancy support program during COVID-19.
OAK STREET HEALTH: (MEDICARE)
   A network of value-based primary care centers serving nearly 80,000 adults on Medicare. It rapidly developed and deployed a remote care program that includes telehealth visits, COVID-19 resources, and support for the social determinants of health. It reported a 51% reduction in hospital admissions and 46% reduction in emergency department visits. It mainly serves patients on Medicare Advantage plans.

IORA HEALTH: (MEDICARE):

A well-established PCP provider network that transformed quickly to non–visit-based care via restructuring of teams, systems, and processes.

CHENMED: (MEDICARE):

Also, a rapidly growing network of primary care practices focused on the needs of older adults with complex medical and psychosocial conditions. It also pivoted from 90% in-center to 95% telemedicine appointments in just 1 week in February 2020.

ONE MEDICAL: (DIRECT CARE PROVIDER)

A membership-based, direct primary care platform targeting working-age adults with '24/7 seamless digital health and as needed in office care' introduced a virtual health offering at the start of the pandemic, including virtual psychotherapy, respiratory symptom triage.

SUMMARY

It is a sad commentary that in a country with the wealth of the United States such significant disparities in health care not only exist but may be increasing. The COVID-19 pandemic has only served to magnify the extent of the disparity both from the difference in the incidence of the disease between white and non-white populations as well as the difference in mortality between these groups. Significant distrust continues to exist among many in the underserved population who feel they have been left out. The emergency room continues to be the default provider for many as the availability of primary care is limited in many communities. Disparity in incidence and mortality between white and non-white populations exists in the spectrum of thoracic surgery diseases including chronic obstructive pulmonary disease, lung transplantation, lung cancer, and esophageal cancer. These differences are clearly multifactorial at the individual, health care system, and socio-political level. Finally, it is incumbent on thoracic surgeons to understand the complexities of health disparities and how it impacts the care we deliver. Furthermore, we must look for opportunities to intervene and mitigate disparities. Now more than ever we need to find a way to make health care accessible to all and provide the highest quality of care with empathy and compassion.

DISCLOSURE

The authors have nothing to disclose.

REFERENCES

1. D-to-D slashed 85% in seven weeks. ED Manag 2009;21(8):90–1.
2. Moskop JC, Sklar DP, Geiderman JM, et al. Emergency department crowding. Part 1. Concept, causes, and moral consequences. Ann Emerg Med 2009;53(5):605–11.
3. Comprehensive emergency department and inpatient changes improve emergency department patient satisfaction, reduce bottlenecks that delay admissions. Available at: http://www.innovations. ahrq.gov/content.aspx?id=1757. Accessed May 25, 2021.
4. Relationship between racial disparities in ED wait times. Available at: https://www.sciencedirect.com/ science/article/abs/pii/S0735675715007445. Accessed May 25, 2021.
5. Changes in health coverage by race and ethnicity since the ACA, 2010-2018 Samantha Artiga, Kendal Orgera and Anthony Damico. KFF.org.
6. Changes at community health centers, and how patients are benefiting results from the Commonwealth Fund National survey of federally qualified health centers, 2013–2018. Available at: https:// www.commonwealthfund.org/publications/issue-bri efs/2019/aug/changes-at-community-health-center s-how-patients-are-benefiting. Accessed October 26, 2021.
7. Community Health Centers and the Affordable Care Act: increasing access to affordable, cost effective, high quality care. Available at: HRSA.gov. Accessed May 24, 2021.
8. Sentell T, Braun KL. Low health literacy, limited English proficiency, and health status in Asians, Latinos, and other racial/ethnic groups in California. J Health Commun 2012;17 Suppl 3(Suppl 3):82–99.
9. NCI Surveillance, Epidemiology, and End Results Program (SEER) database. Available at: https://seer. cancer.gov/statfacts/html/disparities.html. Accessed May 25, 2021.
10. Medicare Hospital readmissions among minority populations. Available at: https://www.cms.gov/ About-CMS-Agency-Information/OMH/Downloads/ OMH_Dwnld-MedicareHospitalRead missionsAmongMinorityPopulations.pdf. Accessed May 24, 2021.
11. Affordable Care Act. Available at: https://en. wikipedia.org/wiki/Affordable_Care_Act. Accessed May 25, 2021.
12. National federation of independent business vs Sebelius. Available at: https://en.wikipedia.org/wiki/ National_Federation_of_Independent_Business_v._ Sebelius. Accessed May 26, 2021.
13. 3 status of state action on the Medicaid expansion decision. San Francisco, CA: Henry J. Kaiser Family Foundation; 2020. Available at: https://www.

kff.org/health-reform/stateindicator/state-activity-around-expanding-medicaid-under-the-affordable-care-act. Accessed May 26, 2021.

14. Number of U.S. Retail Health Clinics Will Surpass 2,800 by 2017, Accenture Forecasts - Accenture Newsroom". Available at: newsroom.accenture.com. Accessed May 26, 2021.

15. KFF health tracking poll (conducted February 13-18, 2020. Available at: https://www.accessonemedcard.com/wp-content/uploads/2020/12/AccessOne-Patient-Finance-Survey-2020.pdf Accessed October 26, 2021.

16. Surprise Medical Bills: new protections for consumers take effect in 2022. Available at: https://www.kff.org/private-insurance/fact-sheet/surprise-medical-bills-new-protections-for-consumers-take-effect-in-2022/. Accessed October 26, 2021

17. Chaudhry SI, Herrin J, Phillips C, et al. Racial disparities in health literacy and access to care among patients with heart failure. J Card Fail 2011;17(2): 122–7.

18. Kutner M., Greenburg E., Jin Y., et al. The health literacy of America's adults: results from the 2003 National assessment of adult Illiteracy. Available at: http://nces.ed.gov/pubsearch/pubsinfo.asp?pubid=2006483. Accessed September 29, 2008.

19. Jang Y, Kim MT. Limited english proficiency and health service use in Asian Americans. J Immigr Minor Health 2019;21(2):264–70.

20. Sentell T, Braun KL. Low health literacy limited English proficiency, and health status in Asians, Latinos, and other racial/ethnic groups in California. J Health Commun 2012;17(Suppl 3):82–99.

21. CDC National Center for Health Statistics analysis of US Census Bureau's Household Pulse Survey. Available at: https://www.cdc.gov/nchs/covid19/pulse/reduced-access-to-care.htm. Accessed May 26, 2021.

22. Passel JS, Cohn D. Pew Hispanic Center: Pew Research Center Social and Demographic Trends. U.S. population projections 2005-2050. Pew Research Center Publications, Washington, DC, 2008.

23. Smedley BD, Stith AY, Nelson AR, editors. Unequal treatment: confronting racial and ethnic disparities in healthcare. Washington, DC: National Academy Press; 2003.

24. Greenwald AG, McGhee DE, Schwarz JL. Measuring individual differences in implicit cognition: the implicit association test. J Pers Soc Psychol 1998;74(6):1464–80.

25. van Ryn M. Research on the provider contribution to race/ethnicity disparities in medical care. Med Care 2002;40(1 Suppl):I140–51.

26. Armstrong K, Rose A, Peters N, et al. Distrust of the health care system and self-reported health in the United States. J Gen Intern Med 2006;21(4):292–7.

27. Syed ST, Gerber BS, Sharp LK. Traveling towards disease: transportation barriers to health care access. J Community Health 2013;38(5):976–93.

Social Disparities in Lung Cancer Risk and Screening

Vignesh Raman, MD, MHS[a],*, Valeda Yong, MD[b], Cherie P. Erkmen, MD[c], Betty C. Tong, MD, MHS[a]

KEYWORDS

- Lung cancer • Screening • Health disparities • Social disparities • Smoking • Risk

KEY POINTS

- The comparative incidence of lung cancer in younger women is increasing relative to men.
- Black people, especially men, seem to be more susceptible to lung cancer even though they smoke less and for a shorter duration compared with White people.
- Individuals in urban neighborhoods are likely experiencing more toxic exposure compared with their rural counterparts and are more likely to develop lung cancer.
- People of lower socioeconomic status or with government-based insurance are more likely to be diagnosed with lung cancer and are more likely to have limited access to screening.
- There are disparities in provider knowledge and belief in lung cancer screening, as well as eligibility for screening.

Lung cancer is the leading cause of mortality related to cancer in the United States and globally.[1] The American Cancer Society estimates that in 2021, about 235,760 new cases of lung cancer will be diagnosed in the United States alone and that about 131,880 people will die from it.[2] The all-stage 5-year survival of non–small cell lung cancer is estimated to be about 25%.[3] However, not all groups of individuals are diagnosed with lung cancer equally.[4] Similarly, there are inequities in patients' access to lung cancer screening and therefore diagnosis as well as with treatment and outcomes. Disadvantaged groups include those who are in developing countries, live in rural areas, have government insurance, have lower income, and are racial and ethnic minorities. In this chapter, the authors examine the disparities experienced by these groups in lung cancer incidence, risk, and diagnosis via screening.

LUNG CANCER INCIDENCE AND RISK
Disparities in Incidence

There are numerous inequities in the incidence of lung cancer in the general population. There are disparities, for instance, in the incidence of lung cancer based on geography. In a study of the GLOBOCAN data from 2012, Cheng and colleagues examined the association of lung cancer incidence and the Human Development Index (HDI), which is a metric of how "developed" a country is considered.[4] They found that lung cancer incidence was highest in countries with a very high HDI and lowest in low-HDI countries (42.2 vs 7.9 in 100,000 for men and 21.8 vs 3.1 in women). Further, men in Central and Eastern Europe had the highest incidence rate, whereas women in North America and Northern Europe had the highest incidence. In addition to regions in the world, there are also disparities in lung cancer incidence

^a Division of Cardiovascular and Thoracic Surgery, Duke University Medical Center, 2301 Erwin Road, Durham, NC 27710, USA; ^b Surgery, Temple University Hospital, 3401 N. Broad Street, Zone C, 4th Floor, Philadelphia, PA 19140, USA; ^c Thoracic Medicine and Surgery, Temple University Hospital, Philadelphia, PA, USA
* Corresponding author.
E-mail address: vignesh.raman@duke.edu
Twitter: @vigneshr11 (V.R.); @ValedaYongMD (V.Y.)

Thorac Surg Clin 32 (2022) 23–31
https://doi.org/10.1016/j.thorsurg.2021.09.011

based on the rurality of patients in the United States. In a study of the Illinois state cancer registry from 1998 to 2002, McLafferty and colleagues found the risk of lung cancer higher in highly urbanized areas, even after controlling for age, race, and access to health care, although the study did not adjust for smoking status.[5]

There is also an increasing inequity in the incidence of lung cancer by sex. In a study of the North American Association of Central Cancer Registries (NAACR) spanning 1995 to 2014, Jemal and colleagues found that female-to-male incidence ratios increased among non-Hispanic White people in the 30 to 49 years age group with a similar trend in Hispanic people.[6] Racioethnic minorities also experience disparities in lung cancer incidence. Black people continue to have higher relative incidence rates of lung cancer even though lung cancer incidence has declined among all racioethnic groups.[7] The age-adjusted incidence rate of lung cancer is about 32% higher in African Americans compared with European Americans.[8] In a study of the National Lung Screening Trial (NLST) cohort, Juon and colleagues found that Black patients had a higher rate of diagnosis (4.3 vs 3.9%) compared with White patients, including a higher odds of lung cancer diagnosis after adjustment for race, smoking status, and occupational exposures (odds ratio [OR] 1.24; 95% confidence interval [CI] 1.01–1.54).[9] Among men, Black men have the highest incidence rates (104.5 per 100,000).[10] Black women who never smoked also have significantly higher incidence rates compared with women of European descent.[11]

Insurance status has also been associated with lung cancer risk. In a study of the Michigan Cancer Registry between 1996 and 1997, Bradley and coworkers reported that women on Medicaid and younger than 65 years had greater than a 4-fold higher incidence of lung cancer compared with women not on Medicaid.[12] Similarly, men younger than 65 years on Medicaid had a 5-fold higher incidence of lung cancer compared with those not on Medicaid. In older patients, Medicaid was still associated with a higher incidence of lung, colon, and cervical cancer. As an extension, socioeconomic status has also been implicated in incidence. Hastert and colleagues examined the association between socioeconomic status and cancer incidence and mortality in patients from the VITamins and Lifestyle (VITAL) study in 2000 to 2002.[13] They found that the lowest quintile of socioeconomic status was associated with higher lung cancer incidence compared with the highest quintile (hazard ratio [HR] 2.2; 95% CI 1.69–2.90), an association that persisted following adjustment for individual education and household income.

However, this study did not adjust for smoking status and race/ethnicity.

Disparities in Risk

There is a complicated relationship between disparities in risk factors for lung cancer and disparities in incidence and outcomes. Smoking is the best understood risk factor for lung cancer. There are both geographic and sociodemographic differences in smoking rates in the United States. Although the overall prevalence of any tobacco use in the United States is approximately 20.8%, rates are higher in the Midwest and South as compared with the Northeast or West. Lung cancer incidence also parallels tobacco use. For instance, lung cancer incidence is higher in Kentucky (smoking prevalence of 30%) than in California (smoking prevalence of 14%).[4]

There are also different rates of smoking between men and women and among racioethnic groups. More men (26.2%) than women (15.7%) use tobacco products in general, with a higher relative proportion of men using combustible products and cigarettes in particular. American Indian/Alaska Natives have the highest rates of cigarette smoking (20.9%) and Asian, non-Hispanic Americans have the lowest (7.2%).

Smoking also has differential effects on carcinogenesis in Black and White populations. For instance, Black people diagnosed with lung cancer are more likely to smoke less and start smoking later in life compared with White people, suggesting that Black people might be more susceptible to the effects of tobacco.[8] However, there is also evidence that lung cancer risk increases more with duration of smoking than quantity of tobacco consumption,[14] with the caveat that even after controlling for both tobacco consumption and smoking duration, Black people are more likely to be diagnosed with lung cancer than White people.[15] Further, Black people are more likely to use menthol cigarettes compared with White people (70%–85% vs 20%–30%), and some studies indicate that menthol cigarettes are associated with lower smoking cessation, although the literature is largely equivocal.[8,16–18]

Besides race, tobacco consumption is also associated with socioeconomic status. Adults in low-income brackets are 2 times more likely to smoke.[19] Siahpush and colleagues found that individuals in poverty smoked for a median of 40 years, whereas those with a family income at least 3 times greater than poverty level smoked for a median of 22 years.[20] Within these low-income neighborhoods, there are more tobacco retailers and targeted advertising campaigns from tobacco companies.[19,21] Historically, the tobacco industry has targeted women of low socioeconomic status through coupons, discounts, and creating brands that appeal to women.[19,22] In addition, adults without a high school diploma are 2 to 3 times more likely to smoke than those with a college degree.[19,20]

There is also evidence that other risks for lung cancer, including air pollution, industrial toxins, and radon, are disproportionately found in working-class communities.[23–30] Asbestos and radon exposure are also overwhelmingly seen in underserved and disabled populations.[31–33] These populations often lack awareness and resources for testing and mitigation.[33] Smoking and radon have a synergistic effect, and radon is the leading cause of lung cancer in never-smokers.[32] It is also the second most common cause of lung cancer in the United States.[32] Similarly, lung cancer risk is 5 times more likely with asbestos exposure.[33] Asbestos exposure can be seen in houses built before 1975, and these houses are considered substandard living situations. Low-income people, people of color, and people with disabilities are more likely to live in inadequate housing, which includes those with asbestos.[33] Of note, individuals with an income less than $25,000 are 4 times more likely to live in inadequate housing than higher-income individuals, African Americans are twice as likely to live in inadequate housing compared with White Americans, and disabled individuals are 1.4 times as likely to live in inadequate housing compared with abled individuals.[33] In addition, air pollution also increases lung cancer risk, and the International Agency for Research termed biomass smoke a probable carcinogen (Group 2a) and coal as carcinogenic for humans (Group 1).[34] These environmental factors further contribute to the increased incidence of lung cancer in Black people and people with socioeconomic deprivation.[23–30]

Limitations

There are numerous limitations in studies examining disparities in lung cancer incidence. For one, most studies are methodologically limited and do not adjust for important risk factors, such as smoking, toxic exposures, and other covariates, which makes it challenging to draw definitive lessons from them. Another complicating factor is the interplay between various disparities. For instance, racial minority groups often also experience socioeconomic deprivation. As an example, compared with White people, minorities in the middle class are more likely to face unemployment.[35] Most studies examining disparities do not meaningfully model the interactions between these variables. Further, there are potential disparities that have not been analyzed. Inequities experienced by the LGBTQ community, for instance, remain uncharacterized, probably in large part because information about sexual orientation and gender identity are self-reported and not historically documented in medical records. Some groups, as those who are undocumented or uninsured, are similarly poorly understood.

LUNG CANCER SCREENING

The incidence of lung cancer is predicated on diagnosis. The introduction of lung cancer screening (LCS) via low-dose computed tomography (LDCT) following the NLST in 2013 theoretically offers a mechanism to increase the detection of lung cancer in people with risk factors.[36] The NLST enrolled 53,454 participants who were 55 to 74 years of age, had 30 pack-years or greater smoking history, and were either current or former smokers who had stopped within 15 years. Patients were randomized to either annual chest X ray (CXR) or annual LDCT. The study found that more lung cancers were diagnosed with LDCT compared with CXR, including a higher fraction of early stage cancers (50% vs 31% stage I). Further, lung cancer mortality decreased by 20% with LCS and overall mortality by 6.7%. Following the NLST, several guidelines, including those by the US Preventative Services Task Force (USPSTF), began recommending LCS.

A more recent landmark trial, NELSON, was conducted in Netherlands and Belgium and enrolled 15,789 people aged 50 to 75 years, with a smoking history of either more than 15 cigarettes a day for more than 25 years or more than 10 cigarettes a day for more than 30 years.[37] Screening with LDCT, compared with no screening, demonstrated a 24% decrease in lung cancer mortality after 10 years of screening. Despite the overwhelming evidence in favor of lung cancer screening, however, only an estimated 3.9% of screen-eligible patients undergo LCS.[38,39] Further, lung cancer screening guidelines may also exclude people who are at risk for lung cancer, propagating inequities in the diagnosis of lung cancer.

Geographic Disparities

Similar to lung cancer incidence, geography affects LCS occurrence. For instance, patients in rural areas are less likely to have access to LCS programs. In a geospatial exploratory study, Martin and coworkers analyzed the presence of LDCT facilities in areas with high adult smoking rates in

Virginia and found that in rural counties, especially in southwest Virginia, only 2 LDCT facilities existed.[40] A study mapping the distance between US smokers and LDCT facilities using census tract data showed that there was an inverse relationship between population density and distance to an LDCT facility, with significant inter- and intrastate variability.[41] Tailor and colleagues showed that in a study of the US Medicare fee-for-service population, there is geographic variation in the proportion of people who are estimated to be eligible for LCS.[42] Moreover, there were also geographic differences in the proportion of these people who received screening studies. Of the screen-eligible patients who underwent LCS, rates were highest in the Northeast and lowest in the South.

Systemic and Societal Disparities

There are several inequities in health policy and guidelines that decrease access to lung cancer screening. For one, the development of an LCS program requires significantly more logistical effort compared with other screening modalities. LCS is the only cancer screening in America that mandates a shared decision-making visit, for instance.[43] In order to be eligible for CMS reimbursement for LCS, data submission to a national registry is mandatory, and this requires cataloging of more than 40 required data fields.[44] Although the reimbursement criteria were designed to ensure patients receive high-quality lung cancer screening, the logistical requirements of implementation can be challenging. Few centers have staff who can dedicate time or resources to developing shared decision-making programs or enter data into the database.[45,46] As a result, smaller centers may be less likely to develop LCS programs, which in turn heightens the disparities in access based on geography as described earlier.

Another potential barrier to equitable screening is the variability in guidelines about eligibility. For instance, the American College of Chest Physicians[47] recommends screening in people aged 55 to 77 years, whereas the Canadian Task Force on Preventive Health Care[48] recommends screening only up to the age of 74 years. The USPSTF recently updated its guidelines to recommend screening patients between the ages of 50 and 80 years.[49,50] Further, there is variation in the smoking history that prompts a screening recommendation, with guidelines ranging from requiring at least 30 pack-years of current or recent smoking to 20 pack-year history or a combination of smoking history and calculated model-based risk.[51] The different guidelines about eligibility for LCS have the potential to sow confusion on the part of patients and referring providers alike and carry the risk of screening without reimbursement.

Provider-Level Disparities

Successful lung cancer screening is also hindered by inequities at the level of the care provider. One major barrier is the provider's lack of understanding of and belief in LCS. Only 36% of primary care physicians surveyed in South Carolina were aware that LCS should be performed every year, and 63% were unsure if Medicare reimbursed the service.[52] In this study, 38% of providers were not even sure if an LDCT facility was available within their vicinity. Most of the providers were unsure about LCS guidelines. Another survey of primary care clinicians reported that only 56% of providers planned to refer patients for LCS and only 10% had a formal LCS program in their practice.[53] In another study, providers were more likely to refer patients with advanced breast cancer to oncologists compared with patients with advanced lung cancer.[54] Primary care providers were also more likely to know that chemotherapy improves survival in breast cancer than that it similarly improves survival in lung cancer, suggesting bias and lack of knowledge about lung cancer can further diminish access to appropriate care for people with lung cancer. Given the reliance on primary care providers to refer patients for appropriate LCS, the lack of knowledge about LCS is an inherent barrier to effective implementation of screening. This may, in part, explain why fewer than 20% of screen-eligible individuals get LCS.[55–58]

Further, it has been shown that providers exhibit bias that influences their ability and willingness to provide equitable care for patients.[59] For instance, in a study of 18 non-Black medical oncologists and 112 Black patients, oncologists with greater implicit racial bias, as measured by an implicit bias instrument weeks before interactions, had shorter interactions that were also rated as less patient-centered and supportive by patients and observers.[60] Implicit bias was also associated with less patient confidence in the recommended treatment and greater difficulty in completing them. In a survey-based study of 103 patients visiting oncology clinics, Black patients reported lower postvisit trust in physicians compared with White patients.[61] Further, Black patients found physicians' communication less informative, less supportive, and less partnering compared with White patients. Such provider bias is likely to lead to less therapeutic relationships between providers and patients and is likely to also inform how providers refer patients for LCS.

Individual Barriers

There are several disparities at the level of individual patients that reduce access to LCS. As described earlier, patients' lack of trust in providers can affect their willingness to undergo recommended treatments. In a study by Penner and colleagues, patients who interacted with providers with higher implicit racial bias experienced more difficulty in completing recommended treatment.[60] Patients with lung cancer also experience greater stigma related to smoking and are likely to blame themselves.[62,63] Fatalism about lung cancer also curbs effective LCS, with about half of current smokers in a study equating a lung cancer diagnosis with a death sentence.[64]

One of the greatest disparities in access to LCS is race. In the NLST, only 4.4% of the cohort was Black, even though Black people comprise 12.3% of the population in the United States.[36] In addition, a post hoc analysis of the NLST data showed a greater mortality reduction in Black compared with White registrants (HR 0.61; 95% CI 0.37–1.01 vs HR 0.86; 95% CI 0.75–0.98),[38] even though Black men were significantly less likely to undergo surgical resection for screen-detected Stage IA NSCLC[65] among Black and White men and women. Screening programs with a higher proportion of minoritized individuals have shown both a higher percentage of current smokers and a higher proportion of positive LDCT scans compared with the NLST cohort.[66]

Black people are also more likely to be diagnosed with lung cancer at an earlier age compared with White people. In a Surveillance, Epidemiology, and End Results study of 468,403 patients, Annangi and colleagues found that age-adjusted incidence rates for lung cancer were higher in African Americans compared with White individuals, with the highest difference noted for people aged 50 to 54 years.[67] In a study of the National Health Interview Survey, Han and colleagues reported that a higher proportion of Black people were ineligible for screening at younger (15.6%) and older (14.2%) ages compared with White people (4.8% and 10.8%, respectively).[68] Other studies have found that non-Black patients were 50% to 90% more likely to meet criteria for LCS than Black patients.[69,70] Further, as characterized earlier, there is evidence that Black people are more susceptible to lung cancer even with less tobacco consumption compared with White individuals. The USPSTF recently liberalized its lung cancer screening recommendations to include patients between the age of 50 to 80 years and who have smoked 20 pack-years, and many have lauded these changes as one way to help reduce disparities in risk that may exist among different racioethnic groups.

Insurance and socioeconomic status also drive inequities in lung screening. In a study of 438 screen-eligible patients in Indiana, Carter-Harris and colleagues found people with government insurance were less likely to intend to undergo screening compared with those with private insurance (52% vs 70%).[71] People in the lowest tertile of income (<$25,000) were also less likely to intend to undergo LCS (48% vs 58%). Low-income people often depend on Medicaid, and the lack of Medicaid expansion in some states will likely worsen socioeconomic disparities in access to LCS, especially because more than half of patients who qualify for LCS are estimated to have Medicaid or be uninsured.[39] Finally, patients infected with human immunodeficiency virus (HIV) have about a 52% increased risk of lung cancer compared with the general population, likely due to immunosuppressive therapies and potentially oncogenic properties of HIV infection.[72] LCS can provide a similar mortality reduction in this population compared with the general population.[73]

Limitations

The literature examining lung cancer screening disparities is riddled with the same limitations as that examining incidence. The interactions between race, geography, and socioeconomic status are not well characterized in most studies, which is a significant methodological limitation. Many studies also do not offer adjustment for confounding by smoking status or other toxic exposures. Disparities potentially present in LGBTQ + individuals have not been examined. One of the biggest limitations is that although the NLST and NELSON have both suggested a greater mortality reduction in women compared with men from LCS, there is scant literature examining potential inequities in women's access to screening and successful screening.

Future Directions

There remains much work to be done to address the inequities in diagnosis of lung cancer. Perhaps most paramount is the need to address the risk factors for smoking and the disparities in smoking and smoking cessation. Smoking cessation programs should be customized to communities at higher risk of smoking: those who face economic deprivation, live in rural areas, and Black men. LCS programs also need to be tailored to communities at higher risk for lung cancer. Programs specifically targeting Black people, rural communities, and those earning lower income need to be developed. In order to address rural communities, mobile LDCT units with telehealth-based smoking cessation and shared decision-making visits may have to be devised to bring screening to the communities. Informational tools to increase awareness of lung cancer and LCS should also be tailored to communities at higher risk. At the provider level, bias training should be instituted to ensure equitable care is provided to patients. Informational campaigns targeting primary care providers should be launched to create awareness about LCS. Empathy-based communication that destigmatizes lung cancer needs to be emphasized.[74] Policy changes should be instituted as well. Although the relaxation of USPSTF guidelines to include patients who are younger and who have smoked less does address some disparities, more work remains. For instance, up to 46% of lung cancers are diagnosed in former smokers beyond 15 years of cessation.[75] Guidelines also do not acknowledge the disparities in lung cancer incidence and diagnosis in minority groups. Medicaid should be expanded to cover LCS. Future clinical trials should also seek to enroll more diverse patients so we can better understand the differential effects of interventions on communities at higher risk.

SUMMARY

Within the context of limitations, there is still abundant evidence that significant disparities exist in the incidence and screening of lung cancer. The comparative incidence of lung cancer in younger women, for instance, is increasing relative to men. Black people, especially men, seem to be more susceptible to lung cancer even though they smoke less and later in life compared with White people. People who live in urban areas likely experience more toxic exposures and are more likely to develop lung cancer compared with those who live in rural areas. People with lower socioeconomic status or who have government-based insurance are also more likely to be diagnosed with lung cancer. Similarly, access to lung cancer screening is limited to those who are on government insurance, who face economic deprivation, and who live in rural areas. Although Black people are more likely to be diagnosed earlier in life with lung cancer, guidelines have largely not accommodated this disparity and Black people are less likely to be eligible for or undergo lung screening compared with White people. Providers also exhibit implicit racial bias that can negatively affect the care of minoritized groups with implications for screening. Many primary care providers do not know about LCS guidelines, and CMS requirements mount a logistical challenge to most institutions to develop lung screening programs. The sum of these factors, among others yet uncharacterized, likely explains why only 4% of eligible patients receive lung cancer screening. Many limitations have been identified in the literature to address in future research into disparities as well as concrete action that can be taken to mitigate disparities so that people can receive equitable screening for lung cancer.

CLINICS CARE POINTS

- Smoking cessation programs should be customized to the populations at higher risk of smoking, such as low-income, rural, and minority communities.
- Lung cancer screening programs need to be tailored to communities at higher risk of developing lung cancer, such as those targeting Black individuals, rural communities, and low-income individuals.
- To address rural communities, mobile lung cancer screening units with telehealth-based smoking cessation and shared decision-making visits should be created.
- Informational tools to increase awareness of lung cancer and screening should be targeted to high-risk communities.
- Providers should undergo bias and empathy-based training to ensure equitable patient care and destigmatize lung cancer.
- Policy changes, such as expanding Medicaid to cover lung cancer screening, should be made.

DISCLOSURE

The authors have nothing to disclose.

REFERENCES

1. Bray F, Ferlay J, Soerjomataram I, et al. Global cancer statistics 2018: GLOBOCAN estimates of incidence and mortality worldwide for 36 cancers in 185 countries. CA Cancer J Clin 2018;68(6): 394–424.
2. Lung Cancer Statistics | How Common is Lung Cancer? [Internet]. Available at: https://www.cancer.org/cancer/lung-cancer/about/key-statistics.html. Accessed January 10, 2021.

3. Lung Cancer Survival Rates | 5-year survival rates for lung cancer [Internet]. Available at: https://www.cancer.org/cancer/lung-cancer/detection-diagnosis-staging/survival-rates.html. Accessed January 10, 2021.

4. Cheng T-YD, Cramb SM, Baade PD, et al. The international epidemiology of lung cancer: latest trends, disparities, and tumor characteristics. J Thorac Oncol 2016;11(10):1653–71.

5. McLafferty S, Wang F. Rural reversal? Cancer 2009; 115(12):2755–64.

6. Jemal A, Miller KD, Ma J, et al. Higher lung cancer incidence in young women than young men in the United States. N Engl J Med 2018;378(21): 1999–2009.

7. Richards TB, Henley SJ, Puckett MC, et al. Lung cancer survival in the United States by race and stage (2001-2009): Findings from the CONCORD-2 study. Cancer 2017;123(S24):5079–99.

8. Ryan BM. Lung cancer health disparities. Carcinogenesis 2018;39(6):741–51.

9. Juon H-S, Hong A, Pimpinelli M, et al. Racial disparities in occupational risks and lung cancer incidence: analysis of the National Lung Screening Trial. Prev Med 2021;143:106355.

10. Underwood JM, Townsend JS, Tai E, et al. Racial and regional disparities in lung cancer incidence. Cancer 2012;118(7):1910–8.

11. Thun MJ, Hannan LM, Adams-Campbell LL, et al. Lung cancer occurrence in never-smokers: an analysis of 13 cohorts and 22 cancer registry studies. PLoS Med 2008;5(9):e185.

12. Bradley CJ, Given CW, Roberts C. Disparities in cancer diagnosis and survival. Cancer 2001;91(1): 178–88.

13. Hastert TA, Beresford SAA, Sheppard L, et al. Disparities in cancer incidence and mortality by area-level socioeconomic status: a multilevel analysis. J Epidemiol Community Health 2015; 69(2):168–76.

14. Lubin JH, Caporaso N, Wichmann HE, et al. Cigarette smoking and lung cancer: modeling effect modification of total exposure and intensity. Epidemiol Camb Mass 2007;18(5):639–48.

15. Haiman CA, Stram DO, Wilkens LR, et al. Ethnic and racial differences in the smoking-related risk of lung cancer. N Engl J Med 2006;354(4):333–42.

16. Accessed January 11, 2021 Menthol and Cigarettes | Smoking & Tobacco Use | CDC [Internet]. 2020. Available at: https://www.cdc.gov/tobacco/basic_information/tobacco_industry/menthol-cigarettes/index.html.

17. Villanti AC, Collins LK, Niaura RS, et al. Menthol cigarettes and the public health standard: a systematic review. BMC Public Health 2017;17(1):983.

18. Alexander LA, Trinidad DR, Sakuma K-LK, et al. Why we must continue to investigate menthol's role in the African American smoking paradox. Nicotine Tob Res 2016;18(Suppl 1):S91–101.

19. Available at: https://www.cdc.gov/tobacco/disparities/low-ses/index.htm. Accessed September 15, 2021.

20. Siahpush M, Singh GH, Jones PR, et al. Racial/ethnic and socioeconomic variations in duration of smoking: results from 2003, 2006 and 2007 tobacco use supplement of the current population surveyexternal icon. J Public Health 2009;32(2):210–8.

21. Yu D, Peterson NA, Sheffer MA, et al. Tobacco outlet density and demographics: analysing the relationships with a spatial regression approach. Public Health 2010;124(7):412–6.

22. Brown-Johnson CG, England LJ, Glantz SA, et al. Tobacco industry marketing to low socioeconomic status women in the USA. Tob Control 2014. https://doi.org/10.1136/tobaccocontrol-2013-051224.

23. Benedetti M, Iavarone I, Comba P, et al. Cancer risk associated with residential proximity to industrial sites: a review. Arch Environ Health 2001;56(4): 342–9.

24. Hendryx M, O'Donnell K, Horn K. Lung cancer mortality is elevated in coal-mining areas of Appalachia. Lung Cancer Amst Neth 2008;62(1):1–7.

25. Apelberg BJ, Buckley TJ, White RH. Socioeconomic and racial disparities in cancer risk from air toxics in Maryland. Environ Health Perspect 2005;113(6): 693–9.

26. Perlin SA, Setzer RW, Creason J, et al. Distribution of industrial air emissions by income and race in the United States: an approach using the toxic release inventory. Environ Sci Technol 1995;29(1):69–80.

27. Dockery DW, Pope CA, Xu X, et al. An association between air pollution and mortality in six U.S. cities. N Engl J Med 1993;329(24):1753–9.

28. Luo J, Hendryx M. Environmental carcinogen releases and lung cancer mortality in rural-urban areas of the United States. J Rural Health 2011; 27(4):342–9.

29. Yu M, Tatalovich Z, Gibson JT, et al. Using a composite index of socioeconomic status to investigate health disparities while protecting the confidentiality of cancer registry data. Cancer Causes Control 2014;25(1):81–92.

30. Wong ML, Clarke CA, Yang J, et al. Incidence of non-small-cell lung cancer among California Hispanics according to neighborhood socioeconomic status. J Thorac Oncol 2013;8(3):287–94.

31. Hovanec J, Siemiatycki J, Conway DI, et al. Lung cancer and socioeconomic status in a pooled analysis of case-control studies. PLoS One 2018;13(2): e0192999.

32. Available at: https://www.epa.gov/radon/health-risk-radon. Accessed September 15, 2021.

33. Available at: https://www.apha.org/policies-and-advocacy/public-health-policy-statements/policy-

database/2020/01/10/eliminating-exposure-to-asbestos. Accessed September 15, 2021.

34. Fullerton DG, Bruce N, Gordon SB. Indoor air pollution from biomass fuel smoke is a major health concern in the developing world. Trans R Soc Trop Med Hyg 2008;102(9):843–51.

35. Williams DR, Kontos EZ, Viswanath K, et al. Integrating multiple social statuses in health disparities research: the case of lung cancer. Health Serv Res 2012;47(3pt2):1255–77.

36. Results of initial low-dose computed tomographic screening for lung cancer. N Engl J Med 2013;368(21):1980–91.

37. Koning HJ, van der Aalst CM, Jong PA, et al. Reduced lung-cancer mortality with volume CT screening in a randomized trial. N Engl J Med 2020;382(6):503–13.

38. Haddad DN, Sandler KL, Henderson LM, et al. Disparities in lung cancer screening: a review. Ann Am Thorac Soc 2020;17(4):399–405.

39. Jemal A, Fedewa SA. Lung cancer screening with low-dose computed tomography in the United States-2010 to 2015. JAMA Oncol 2017;3(9):1278–81.

40. Martin AN, Hassinger TE, Kozower BD, et al. Disparities in lung cancer screening availability: lessons from southwest virginia. Ann Thorac Surg 2019;108(2):412–6.

41. Tailor TD, Choudhury KR, Tong BC, et al. Geographic access to ct for lung cancer screening: a census tract-level analysis of cigarette smoking in the United States and driving distance to a CT facility. J Am Coll Radiol 2019;16(1):15–23.

42. Tailor TD, Tong BC, Gao J, et al. Utilization of lung cancer screening in the medicare fee-for-service population. Chest 2020;158(5):2200–10.

43. Decision memo for screening for lung cancer with low dose computed tomography (LDCT) (CAG-00439N). Available at: https://www.cms.gov/medicare-coverage-database/details/nca-decision-memo.aspx?NCAId=274&NcaName=Screening%20for%20Lung%20Cancer%20with%20Low%20Dose%20Computed%20Tomography%20%28LDCT%29&TimeFrame=7&DocType=All&bc=AQAAIAAAAgAAAA%3D%3D. Accessed January, 14 2021.

44. LCSR required data elements [Internet]. ACR Support. Available from: https://nrdrsupport.acr.org/support/solutions/articles/11000041252-lcsr-required-data-elements. Accessed January, 14 2021.

45. Gesthalter YB, Koppelman E, Bolton R, et al. Evaluations of implementation at early-adopting lung cancer screening programs: lessons learned. Chest 2017;152(1):70–80.

46. Carter-Harris L, Gould MK. Multilevel barriers to the successful implementation of lung cancer

screening: why does it have to be so hard? Ann Am Thorac Soc 2017;14(8):1261–5.

47. Screening for lung cancer: CHEST guideline and expert panel report. Available at: http://info.chestnet.org/screening-for-lung-cancer-chest-guideline-and-expert-panel-report. Accessed January, 14 2021.

48. Canadian Task Force on preventive health care | lung cancer. Available at: https://canadiantaskforce.ca/guidelines/published-guidelines/lung-cancer/. Accessed January, 14 2021.

49. US Preventive Services Task Force, Krist AH, Davidson KW, Mangione CM, et al. Screening for lung cancer: US preventive services task force recommendation statement. JAMA 2021;325(10):962.

50. Potter AL, Bajaj SS, Yang C-FJ. The 2021 USPSTF lung cancer screening guidelines: a new frontier. Lancet Respir Med 2021;9(7):689–91.

51. Jaklitsch MT, Jacobson FL, Austin JHM, et al. The American Association for Thoracic Surgery guidelines for lung cancer screening using low-dose computed tomography scans for lung cancer survivors and other high-risk groups. J Thorac Cardiovasc Surg 2012;144(1):33–8.

52. Ersek JL, Eberth JM, McDonnell KK, et al. Knowledge of, attitudes toward, and use of low-dose computed tomography for lung cancer screening among family physicians. Cancer 2016;122(15):2324–31.

53. Volk RJ, Foxhall LE. Readiness of primary care clinicians to implement lung cancer screening programs. Prev Med Rep 2015;2:717–9.

54. Wassenaar TR, Eickhoff JC, Jarzemsky DR, et al. Differences in primary care clinicians' approach to non-small cell lung cancer patients compared with breast cancer. J Thorac Oncol 2007;2(8):722–8.

55. Richards TB, Doria-Rose VP, Soman A, et al. Lung cancer screening inconsistent with U.S. preventive services task force recommendations. Am J Prev Med 2019;56(1):66–73.

56. Tailor TD, Choudhury KR, Tong BC, et al. Geographic access to CT for lung cancer screening: a census tract-level analysis of cigarette smoking in the United States and driving distance to a CT facility. J Am Coll Radiol 2019;16(1):15–23.

57. Narayan AK, Gupta Y, Little BP, et al. Lung cancer screening eligibility and use with low-dose computed tomography: results from the 2018 Behavioral Risk Factor Surveillance System cross-sectional survey. Cancer 2021;127(5):748–56.

58. Zahnd WE, Eberth JM. Lung cancer screening utilization: a behavioral risk factor surveillance system analysis. Am J Prev Med 2019;57(2):250–5.

59. Rivera MP, Katki HA, Tanner NT, et al. Addressing disparities in lung cancer screening eligibility and healthcare access. An official American thoracic

society statement. Am J Respir Crit Care Med 2020;
202(7):e95–112.

60. Penner LA, Dovidio JF, Gonzalez R, et al. The effects
of oncologist implicit racial bias in racially discordant oncology interactions. J Clin Oncol 2016;
34(24):2874–80.

61. Gordon HS, Street RL, Sharf BF, et al. Racial differences in trust and lung cancer patients' perceptions
of physician communication. J Clin Oncol 2006;
24(6):904–9.

62. Borondy Kitts AK. The patient perspective on lung
cancer screening and health disparities. J Am Coll
Radiol 2019;16(4 Part B):601–6.

63. Niederdeppe J, Levy AG. Fatalistic beliefs about
cancer prevention and three prevention behaviors.
Cancer Epidemiol Biomark Prev 2007;16(5):
998–1003.

64. Quaife SL, Marlow LAV, McEwen A, et al. Attitudes
towards lung cancer screening in socioeconomically
deprived and heavy smoking communities: informing screening communication. Health Expect 2017;
20(4):563–73.

65. Balekian AA, Wisnivesky JP, Gould MK. Surgical disparities among patients with stage I lung cancer in
the national lung screening trial. Chest 2019;
155(1):44–52.

66. Pasquinelli MM, Kovitz KL, Koshy M, et al. Outcomes from a minority-based lung cancer screening
program vs the national lung screening trial. JAMA
Oncol 2018;4(9):1291–3.

67. Annangi S, Nutalapati S, Foreman MG, et al. Potential racial disparities using current lung cancer

screening guidelines. J Racial Ethn Health Disparities 2019;6(1):22–6.

68. Han SS, Chow E, Haaf K, et al. Disparities of national
lung cancer screening guidelines in the US population. J Natl Cancer Inst 2020;112(11):1136–42.

69. Japuntich SJ, Krieger NH, Salvas AL, et al. Racial
disparities in lung cancer screening: an exploratory
investigation. J Natl Med Assoc 2018;110(5):
424–7.

70. Li C-C, Matthews AK, Rywant MM, et al. Racial disparities in eligibility for low-dose computed tomography lung cancer screening among older adults with
a history of smoking. Cancer Causes Control 2019;
30(3):235–40.

71. Carter-Harris L, Slaven JE, Monahan PO, et al. Understanding lung cancer screening behavior: racial,
gender, and geographic differences among Indiana
long-term smokers. Prev Med Rep 2018;10:49–54.

72. Robbins HA, Pfeiffer RM, Shiels MS, et al. Excess
cancers among HIV-infected people in the United
States. J Natl Cancer Inst 2015;107(4):dju503.

73. Kong CY, Sigel K, Criss SD, et al. Benefits and
harms of lung cancer screening in HIV-infected individuals with CD4+ cell count at least 500 cells/μl.
AIDS 2018;32(10):1333–42.

74. Banerjee SC, Haque N, Schofield EA, et al.
Oncology care provider training in empathic
communication skills to reduce lung cancer stigma.
Chest 2021;159(5):2040–9.

75. Pinsky PF, Zhu CS, Kramer BS. Lung cancer risk by
years since quitting in 30+ pack year smokers.
J Med Screen 2015;22(3):151–7.

Social Disparities in Lung Cancer

Irmina Elliott, MD, Cayo Gonzalez, BA, Leah Backhus, MD, MPH, Natalie Lui, MD*

KEYWORDS

• Social disparities • Lung cancer disparities • Guideline-concordant treatment for lung cancer

KEY POINTS

- Black patients with lung cancer are less likely to receive guideline-concordant treatment and have worse overall survival than white patients.
- Patients of lower socioeconomic status and those from rural areas are less likely to receive guideline-concordant treatment and have worse overall survival.
- Older patients are less likely to receive guideline-concordant treatment, but when they do, appear to have a survival benefit.
- Female patients with lung cancer have better overall survival than male patients with lung cancer.
- Disparities related to sexual identity and disability have not been well studied.

INTRODUCTION

This article reviews the available literature on racial, sex, sexual identity, age, disability, socioeconomic, and geographic disparities in lung cancer diagnosis, treatment, and outcomes. Data characterizing these disparities primarily come from large national databases, which are well powered to detect survival differences but are not always able to control for relevant cofounders, such as smoking status, comorbidities, detailed histology and stage variables, and details of treatment received. Conversely, studies using smaller single-institution or state databases provide more granular covariate information but have less statistical power. Certain settings, such as Veterans Affairs (VA) hospitals, military hospitals, or data from the Kaiser Permanente system, can be useful in controlling for specific confounders, such as insurance status and access to care. In examining data from these different sources, each with their own strengths and weaknesses, it is evident that social disparities in lung cancer diagnosis, treatment, and outcomes persist. Understanding and ameliorating these disparities is critical to providing appropriate care to patients with lung cancer in the United States.

BODY

Race

Much of the literature on racial disparities in lung cancer has focused on non–small cell lung cancer (NSCLC) in black compared with white patients. Numerous studies with varying methodology (national, regional, and single-institution databases) have demonstrated a survival disadvantage for black patients.

Diagnosis

African Americans and Native Hawaiians have disproportionately higher rates of lung cancer for the same smoking exposure compared with whites.[1] Black communities have historically been exposed to a higher volume of tobacco advertising in both concentration and density; for example, magazines targeted to the black community are 10 times more likely to have cigarette ads than general audience magazines.[2] These targeted tobacco marketing efforts have promoted mentholated cigarettes approximately 70% of the time, resulting in marked differences in use of menthol cigarettes among blacks (estimated at 85% compared with 29% among whites).[3] Menthol alters nicotine metabolism and increases

Department of Cardiothoracic Surgery, Stanford University, 300 Pasteur Dr Falk Cardiovascular Research Building, Stanford, CA 94305-5407, USA
* Corresponding author.
E-mail address: natalielui@stanford.edu

Thorac Surg Clin 32 (2022) 33–42
https://doi.org/10.1016/j.thorsurg.2021.09.009

its bioavailability, which may be associated with more severe levels of addiction.[4] Furthermore, black menthol cigarette smokers have a 12% lower odds of successfully quitting smoking compared with nonmenthol smokers.[5,6]

Survival

Although lung cancer survival rates have improved over time, survival for each stage is worse among black patients compared with white patients, and data extracted from the CONCORD-2 study showed that this disparity is largest when comparing patients with early-stage, presumably treatable, lung cancer.[7] A Surveillance, Epidemiology, and End Results (SEER) analysis found that African American and American Indian patients with stage I NSCLC had worse overall survival compared with Caucasian patients, whereas Asian/Pacific Islander patients had better overall survival.[8] These differences were not present in multivariate analysis that controlled for sex, age, treatment, histology, and stage. A study of patients with stage I NSCLC in the SEER-Medicare database found that black patients were less likely to be treated, were less likely to be treated with surgery alone, and had worse overall survival. However, when comparing within treatment groups, there was no difference in survival by race.[9] This was corroborated in a study of both SEER-Medicare and VA patients with stage I NSCLC, which found that black patients were less likely to receive surgical treatment than white patients. In both databases, overall survival was worse for black patients, but this disparity was eliminated when comparing patients who received the same treatment.[10]

However, this survival disparity has not been documented in small cell lung cancer (SCLC). An SEER review of patients with SCLC found no survival difference by race for stage I, II, or IV patients, and a statistically significant difference for patients with stage III disease, with white patients having the shortest median survival of 12.7 months, compared with 13.6 months in black patients, 13.4 months in Hispanic patients, 13.9 months in Asian patients, and 13.5 months in American Indian patients.[11]

Access to care

One proposed mediator for this survival disparity is unequal access to care as a barrier to receipt of guideline-recommended treatment. For example, a multivariate analysis of patients with lung cancer at Walter Reed Army Medical Center did not find race to be independently associated with worse survival, and the investigators propose that the lack of disparity is explained by equal access to care within the Army health system.[12] Similarly, a study at the University of Maryland Medical Center, where the investigators suggest patients had equal access to care, found that among patients with stage III NSCLC treated with chemoradiation ± surgery, there was no survival difference by race, even though black patients were less likely to receive surgery.[13] Review of stage I/II NSCLC patients in the National Cancer Database (NCDB) found that black patients who were treated at academic centers were more likely to undergo surgery and had improved 3- and 5-year survival compared with black patients treated at community hospitals.[14]

Other studies have demonstrated the persistence of survival disparities despite presumably equal access to care. A single-institution study of patients with NSCLC matched black patients to white patients 1:4 and found worse survival among black patients with stage I, II, and III disease. In multivariate analysis, the survival difference in stage I and II was mitigated by controlling for socioeconomic status (SES), and in stage III disease when controlling for receipt of neoadjuvant therapy.[15] An examination of patients in the California Cancer Registry with stage I/II NSCLC comparing Kaiser members with nonmembers found that black patients were less likely to receive surgery even if they were Kaiser members, demonstrating that access to an integrated health care system does not mitigate this disparity.[16]

Guideline-concordant treatment

The race-based disparity in lung cancer survival is at least in part explained by a disparity in receipt of guideline-concordant treatment, particularly differential rates of surgical resection for early-stage disease. An SEER review of patients with lung cancer during 1995 to 1999 found black patients were 66% less likely to receive timely and appropriate treatment, and black men were half as likely to undergo resection as white men.[17] Another SEER database review found that compared with white patients, black and Hispanic patients were less likely to be offered surgery for stage I NSCLC (adjusted odds ratio [OR] 0.64 and 0.75, respectively).[18] A study of the South Carolina Cancer Registry published in 2008 demonstrated significantly lower rates of resection among black patients (adjusted OR 0.43).[19] A regional study of NSCLC patients in Alabama highlights the intersectionality of race and rurality, identifying urban black patients as less likely to undergo resection (49.3% vs 33.0%, respectively), whereas rural black patients were even less likely to undergo resection (49.8% vs 23.9%, respectively).[20] Despite the lower odds of being offered surgical resection and undergoing said procedure, when black patients actually receive recommended surgical care, their cancer outcomes are comparable to white patients, raising questions of medical distrust and biases as important targets for intervention.[21] Among those patients who do not undergo surgery when offered, black patients are also less likely to receive stereotactic body radiation therapy (SBRT) as another curative option. Although the disparity in surgical treatment has improved in more recent years, the disparity in SBRT use has worsened over time.[22]

An SEER-Medicare study of patients with stage I/II NSCLC who were evaluated by a surgeon within 6 months of diagnosis found a significant surgeon-level difference in the likelihood a black versus white patient being recommended surgical resection, indicating that physician-level bias may play a role. Interestingly, thoracic specialization attenuated this effect.[23] An analysis of the Nationwide Inpatient Sample data demonstrated that black patients had lower risk-adjusted postoperative complication and mortality rates, and Hispanic and Asian patients had lower complication rates.[24] This raises the possibility that nonwhite patients and their physicians may overestimate surgical risk, and fewer "surgically fit" nonwhite patients are offered and undergo resection.

Medical hesitancy

Treatment hesitancy among black patients has been suggested as a mediator of race-based lung cancer disparity. A review of the SEER database identified patients who were recommended surgery but refused; this overall number was low at 1.5%, but nonwhite patients were significantly more likely to refuse surgery (OR 1.95 for black patients, OR 2.03 for other races).[25] Of patients recommended to have surgery for stage I/II NSCLC, 69% of black versus 83% of white patients actually underwent resection.[21] Surveys of minority patients in New York found that factors such as negative surgical beliefs, fatalism, and medical mistrust partially mediate treatment hesitancy among nonwhite patients with lung cancer.[26] Patient and provider biases may contribute to delays in diagnosis, leading to later stage at presentation with potentially devastating impacts on cancer outcomes.

Equal outcomes with equal treatment

Studies have consistently shown that when black patients receive guideline-concordant treatment, they have equivalent survival compared with white patients.[8–10] Thus, efforts to increase rates of guideline-concordant treatment among black patients should be prioritized. Results of a trial conducted at 5 cancer centers to improve compliance with guideline-concordant treatment indicated that with the implementation of a system-based intervention program that included race-specific feedback to clinicians and use of patient navigators, rate of curative-intent treatment increased from 69% to 96% for black patients and from 78% to 95% for white patients.[27] Somewhat reassuringly, a VA study of patients with NSCLC stage I/II found that differences in surgery rates in black compared with white patients have equalized over time, and this is associated with a disappearance in differences in overall and lung cancer–specific survival.[28]

Among patients treated in clinical trials for SCLC, there was no race-based disparity in outcome. Despite a higher rate of factors often associated with worse outcomes, such as poor performance status, lower SES, and history of weight loss, supporting the hypothesis that uniform treatment algorithms, as found in clinical trials, can attenuate survival disparities.[29] The possibility of genetic differences mediating outcome differences in black patients has been postulated, but this has not been supported by genomic data, and rather, is contradicted by the fact that when given the same treatment, survival disparities tend to be mitigated.[30]

Other racial groups

Much of the literature on racial disparity has focused on comparing black and white patients, and comparatively little is known about disparities in lung cancer among other racial groups. Some studies have suggested better survival for Hispanic and Asian patients. For example, a large meta-analysis found that the adjusted risk of death was lower for Hispanics and Asians compared with non-Hispanic whites.[31] Similarly, a single-institution study from the Bronx found Hispanic patients with lung cancer to have improved survival compared with white and black patients, even when adjusting for smoking status.[32]

An SEER-Medicare review found that American Indian and Alaskan Native patients with stage I to IIIA NSCLC have worse aggregate survival when compared with white patients and are more likely to be diagnosed at a later stage and less likely to undergo surgery. However, when controlling for stage and resection, survival differences were no longer significant.[33] An SEER-Medicare review of all lung cancer cases found that American Indians and Alaskan Natives were less likely to undergo resection and had worse survival compared with white patients, and these differences were not explained by slight differences in the distribution of histologic subtypes.[34]

A study examining subgroups of Asian/Pacific Islander populations in California identified significant heterogeneity in histology among subgroups, sex-based differences (perhaps because of sex-based variation in smoking status), and outcomes, and the investigators highlight the need to consider diversity within racial/ethnic groups to appropriately target initiatives to address disparities.[35]

Sex

Research on sex-based differences in lung cancer has revealed that, in general, lung cancer in women is increasing in incidence, and female patients are more likely to be young, have adenocarcinoma histology, and have better median survival. One of the most striking differences in lung cancer epidemiology in women compared with men is the disproportionately high incidence of lung cancer among never or light female smokers.[36] Nonetheless, 80% of female lung cancer is still linked to smoking (compared with more than 90% in men).[36] In addition, as seen in black patients, women are more likely to smoke menthol cigarettes, and some studies have found women are less likely to successfully quit smoking than men.[5]

In the under-50 age group, the nationwide population-based incidence of lung cancer in women now exceeds the incidence among men, and this finding is not fully explained by changes in smoking patterns.[37] A study of the Prostate, Lung, Colorectal, and Ovarian Screening Trial found that hormone replacement therapy (HRT) use was associated with a decreased risk of NSCLC (hazard ratio [HR], 0.8), suggesting that the trend of decreasing prevalence of HRT among postmenopausal women may mirror the increasing lung cancer incidence owing to lowering of a protective effect.[38]

A population-based study of patients with lung cancer in Florida found that women had better median survival than men after controlling for available socioeconomic, clinical, and comorbidity factors.[39] An SEER-Medicare study of patients with stage I/II NSCLC stratified by treatment group (surgery, chemotherapy or radiation, or no treatment) found that women had better survival in each treatment group after controlling for possible confounders, even among patients who were untreated.[40] Similarly, a single-institution series of more than 1000 patients with stage I/II/III NSCLC found female patients to have better survival when controlling for age, stage, and histology. Female patients also appeared to have a better response to neoadjuvant treatment, in that they were more likely to be complete or partial responders.[41] Interestingly, a Society of Thoracic Surgeons Database review published in 2014 found that women have fewer postoperative complications and lower in-hospital and 30-day mortality.[42] A review of the National Inpatient Sample also found female sex to be correlated with lower postoperative morbidity and mortality following lung cancer resection.[24] Whether this short-term advantage may confer improved long-term survival in women remains to be determined.

There are some data to suggest that optimal chemotherapy regimens may differ for male and female patients. For example, a randomized controlled trial of patients with stage IIIB/IV NSCLC found that bevacizumab improved survival when added to paclitaxel/carboplatin, but subset analysis revealed this benefit was seen only in male patients, not female patients.[43] The mechanism of this is unclear, but as the investigators discuss, stratification by sex may be an important factor when evaluating response to chemotherapy in lung cancer.

The underpinnings of the improved outcomes consistently observed in female patients are unknown. Plausible but unproven biologic differences may contribute, such as the interplay of estrogen and hormone receptors in lung cancer, or sex differences in EGFR mutation frequency. Studies of the impact of HRT on lung cancer diagnosis have yielded mixed results. Epidemiologic differences, such as the higher proportion of adenocarcinoma in young female nonsmokers, may also confound survival data.[44]

These sex-based differences in biology and epidemiology complicate the evaluation of possible sex-based disparities. However, an SEER study found that from 1995 to 1999, women with stage I/II NSCLC were 25% less likely to undergo timely surgical resection than men.[17] More current data on the receipt of guideline-concordant treatment by sex are needed to understand if treatment disparities persist. Future investigation of sex-based differences in lung cancer outcomes will require thoughtful consideration of the interplay of biology and disparity.

Sexual Identity

The authors did not identify any literature examining disparities in lung cancer based on sexual identity. The Institute of Medicine has emphasized the importance on the collection of sexual orientation and gender identity data in order to accurately delineate the health disparities that lesbian, gay, bisexual, and transgender people face overall, and this may enable future research on disparities in lung cancer specifically.[45]

Age

Age-based disparities in lung cancer are likely due to the fact that physicians tend to overestimate the risk of treatment for older patients. There may also be a misperception and nihilism that elderly patients are less likely to derive a survival benefit from treatment.

A review of the SEER-Medicare database of patients older than 65 years with lung cancer, including stage I–III and both NSCLC and SCLC, found that increasing age was associated with decreased likelihood of guideline-concordant treatment, which was associated with worse survival. Specifically, patients aged 66 to 69 years were 2.6 times more likely to receive treatment compared with those older than age 80 years, and receipt of guideline-concordant treatment was associated with improved 3-year survival (41% vs 23%).[46] In a study using the NCDB of patients older than the age of 80 years with stage III NSCLC, 63% of patients received no cancer-directed treatment. Patients older than 80 years who received chemoradiation had a 2-year survival of 32%, compared with 17% in those who received no treatment.[47] In an SEER-Medicare review of patients with SCLC (any stage), those older than 85 years were much less likely to receive chemotherapy compared with those 65 to 69 years, but the investigators found that even among patients older than 80 years, chemotherapy was associated with a 6-month improvement in median survival.[48]

Importantly, the literature indicates that when elderly patients receive any cancer-directed treatment at all, they appear to gain a significant survival benefit. As these data are retrospective in nature, it is impossible to determine if older patients who do receive treatment and do well were simply appropriately selected, or whether those who did not receive treatment would have truly benefited. Factors such as frailty, serious medical comorbidities, and patient willingness are among the possible legitimate reasons that elderly patients might decide with their physicians to not pursue cancer therapy. However, overestimation of the risk of treatment and underestimation of possible benefit likely result in underutilization of cancer treatment in this population. In addition, these studies consistently found that among older patients, black patients and those of lower SES were less likely to be treated and/or have worse survival, indicating an aspect of intersectionality in age and racial/socioeconomic disparities.[46,48,49]

Studying these age-based disparities can be challenging, as different age groups appear to be at risk for developing biologically distinct lung cancers. For example, an SEER database review of young patients with lung cancer, defined as those less than 40 years of age, demonstrated that these patients were more likely to be women, to be Asian or Pacific Islanders, to have adenocarcinoma histology, and to have distant metastatic disease. These patients have a high incidence of targetable mutations and have better survival compared with patients with lung cancer overall. The investigators discuss that these findings appear more consistent with a distinct disease process in these young patients, as opposed to a health care disparity.[49]

Disability

There has been little investigation on disparities in the diagnosis, treatment, and survival of lung cancer in patients with and without disabilities in the United States. One study using merged SEER-Medicare data, specifically looking at patients aged 21 to 64 years with stage I lung cancer, found that patients with disabilities underwent surgery at lower rates and had higher lung cancer-specific mortality.[50] However, this survival disparity disappeared when adjusting for receipt of surgery. As the investigators discuss, this study was not able to differentiate between legitimate factors, such as poor physiologic reserve, and inappropriate undertreatment, perhaps because of overestimated surgical risk in patients with disabilities. An alternative interpretation of these data is that those patients with disabilities who are correctly deemed appropriate for surgery have outcomes concordant to those patients without disabilities. Nonetheless, the data suggest that patients with disabilities who are diagnosed with lung cancer are likely undertreated, because of real or perceived surgical increased risk, and this results in increased cancer-specific mortality.[50] Further investigation of this disparity is warranted. As in the case of age disparities, the existing data simply underscore the importance of patient selection independent of bias in determining candidacy for treatment.

Socioeconomic Status

Diagnosis

Several investigators have demonstrated an association between low SES and advanced stage at lung cancer diagnosis. A study of the Metropolitan Detroit Cancer Surveillance System of patients with lung cancer concluded that SES was an independent predictor of stage at diagnosis for lung cancer, with high SES individuals more likely to present with local stage disease when adjusting for race, age, and sex.[51] Two studies of patients within the NCDB as well as a systematic review conducted by the American Thoracic Society similarly reported that uninsured and Medicaid patients were more likely to present with advanced-stage lung cancer compared with privately insured patients.[52–54]

In addition, a study from the Florida Cancer Data System found that patients from less affluent areas were diagnosed with lung cancer at a younger age on average than those from affluent areas (45.3 vs 54.3 years), possibly indicating differences in environmental exposures.[55]

Treatment

Patients of low SES are more likely to receive guideline discordant care. A study of the NCDB found that various SES factors were associated with receipt of guideline discordant treatment for stage I NSCLC. The investigators report that receipt of nonstandard treatment with chemotherapy with or without radiation, as opposed to primary resection, was increased for patients of low income (OR 1.34), low high school graduation rate (OR 1.16), and those with Medicaid or no insurance (OR 1.34). This study found that patients with several SES risk factors have linearly increasing odds of receiving nonstandard treatment.[56] Similar results have been reported using other data sets, including a study of the California Cancer Registry data of patients with stage I NSCLC patients examining low/high poverty neighborhoods, and the Nebraska Cancer Registry for primary localized NSCLC patients, using a composite SES measure (comprising 7 indicator variables that measured education, income, and occupation).[57,58]

There is also disparity in the use of adjuvant therapy following resection in pN1 NSCLC patients; a review of the NCDB demonstrated that patients were less likely to receive multiagent adjuvant chemotherapy if they were uninsured or on Medicaid compared with those patients with all other forms of insurance (OR 1.23).[59]

An NCDB study examining factors associated with treatment refusal for stage IV NSCLC identified several SES variables that were predictive of treatment refusal. The investigators found that factors associated with refusal of radiation included Medicaid or Medicare as primary insurance, uninsured status, low household median income, and lower educational level. Factors associated with chemotherapy refusal were uninsured patients, Medicaid patients, and patients with a high comorbidity index.[60]

Survival

Unsurprisingly, these disparities in diagnosis and treatment appear to translate to a survival disparity for low SES patients with lung cancer. A multivariate analysis of stage I NSCLC patients in the California Cancer Registry data demonstrated a stepwise improvement in survival with increasing SES quintile that was independent of surgery, race, and marital status.[58] This association between SES and survival is supported by several studies using national databases, such as the Nationwide Inpatient Sample and NCDB.[24,61,62]

In patients with pN1 NSCLC, SES factors were independently associated with increased mortality, including lower income (HR, 1.06) or uninsured or Medicaid insurance status (HR, 1.22).[59] Similarly, a study using the NCDB found that factors associated with better survival among limited stage SCLC patients were high income, high education, and private insurance.[63] Interestingly, a study examining stage III or stage IV NSCLC and SCLC patients enrolled in clinical trials found that education did not affect patient survival, suggesting that the protocolization of treatment in the clinical trial setting may ameliorate the SES disparity.[64]

SES is inconsistently defined, and investigators may use indicators such as income, occupation, education level, and insurance status as surrogates. Despite this variety in definition, the literature consistently shows that patients of lower SES are more likely to present at a later stage of disease, receive inferior treatment, and have worse survival.[52,53]

Geographic Location

The literature examining the impact of geographic location on lung cancer suggests a disadvantage for patients living in rural areas.

Diagnosis

Some investigators have hypothesized that because of decreased access to care, rurality might be associated with a later stage at diagnosis. A retrospective cohort study of patients with NSCLC in the Georgia Comprehensive Cancer Registry reported that rural and suburban patients had increased odds of unstaged disease compared with urban patients, which persisted after adjustment for age, gender, race, and tumor grade (suburban OR = 1.23, rural OR = 1.63).[65] However, a study of Medicare patients reported no difference across geographic regions in lung cancer stage at diagnosis.[66] An SEER Database review found that although stage at diagnosis was comparable between rural and urban patients, stage data were more frequently unknown for rural patients than for urban patients and that rural patients had a higher incidence of SCLC cases, likely explained by higher prevalence of smoking in rural areas.[67]

Treatment

There is consistent evidence demonstrating a geographically mediated disparity in lung cancer treatment. A review of the NCDB found that rurality was associated with stage I NSCLC patients undergoing either no treatment or nonstandard treatments.[56] A separate analysis of the NCDB found that rurality was associated with guideline discordant care among patients with stage I NSCLC.[68] A study of the receipt of NSCLC treatment among black and white Medicare beneficiaries in Alabama using the Alabama State Cancer Registry highlighted the intersectionality of race and geography; among patients with stages I–IIIA NSCLC, black patients with Medicare residing in urban counties had 45% lower odds of undergoing surgery than urban white patients, and black Medicare patients residing in rural counties were 67% less likely to receive surgery compared with white rural patients.[20] A review of the NCDB found that patients with pN1 NSCLC were less likely to receive multiagent adjuvant chemotherapy if they lived in a rural area.[59] A separate NCDB analysis showed no association between geography and treatment refusal, suggesting that this treatment disparity is not mediated by patient preference.[60]

Although most work on rurality has focused on patient geography, a study across several institutions in a community-based health care system in the Mississippi Delta region found that care at an urban institution was associated with higher rates of stage-appropriate treatment and improved patient survival for rural patients when compared with rural patients receiving care at rural institutions.[69]

Outcomes

An analysis of the NCDB found that rural patients within each stage of NSCLC diagnosis have a lower overall survival than their urban counterparts. Patients with stage I NSCLC had the greatest absolute difference in overall survival, 11.1 months. In addition, the overall survival was lower for rural compared with nonrural patients who underwent lobectomy for their stage I NSCLC. The overall survival disparity did not persist among those stage I patients who underwent SBRT. Thus, researchers hypothesize that the differences in quality of surgical intervention or postsurgical care may underpin the disparity among rural and urban stage I NSCLC patients who received the same surgical treatment.[68]

An SEER database analysis also found that rural patients with stage I NSCLC had shorter survival compared with urban patients and hypothesized that the survival difference may be explained by surgical care access disparities.[67] An analysis of county level lung cancer mortality data found that mortality was not associated with differences in density of thoracic surgeons or oncologists, but rather may be attributable to availability of primary care.[70] Another aspect of geographic disparity that merits consideration is racial segregation at the population level; an SEER study demonstrated that lung cancer mortality was highest for blacks living in the most segregated counties, regardless of SES.[71] The association between geography and worse lung cancer survival is likely multifactorial and warrants further study.

Taken together, the data indicate many disparities in treatment and survival for rural patients with lung cancer. Challenges in studying these disparities include differences in definitions and coding schemes of rurality, inability of large databases to control for important cofounders, such as smoking prevalence (which has significant geographic variability), and how to best analyze geography when patients may seek care outside of the area in which they live.

SUMMARY

Knowledge of existing social disparities is critical for those who treat patients with lung cancer. Surgeons need to consider these disparities and their own implicit bias when determining who is a candidate for surgery or other treatment. If it is determined that a patient is not a candidate for guideline-concordant treatment, they must ask themselves why, and whether bias has influenced that determination. The health care system must continue efforts to expand access to guideline-concordant care, and as an academic community, they need to support research efforts in this realm to further the understanding of disparities, create interventions to mitigate disparities, and track the evolution of disparities over time.

DISCLOSURES

The authors have no conflicts to disclose.

REFERENCES

1. Haiman CA, Stram DO, Wilkens LR, et al. Ethnic and racial differences in the smoking-related risk of lung cancer. N Engl J Med 2006;354(4):333–42.
2. Primack BA, Bost JE, Land SR, et al. Volume of tobacco advertising in African American markets: systematic review and meta-analysis. Public Health Rep 2007;122(5):607–15.

3. Giovino GA, Villanti AC, Mowery PD, et al. Differential trends in cigarette smoking in the USA: is menthol slowing progress? Tob Control 2015;24(1):28–37.

4. Wickham RJ. The biological impact of menthol on tobacco dependence. Nicotine Tob Res 2020;22(10):1676–84.

5. Smith SS, Fiore MC, Baker TB. Smoking cessation in smokers who smoke menthol and non-menthol cigarettes. Addiction 2014;109(12):2107–17.

6. Smith PH, Assefa B, Kainth S, et al. Use of mentholated cigarettes and likelihood of smoking cessation in the United States: a meta-analysis. Nicotine Tob Res 2020;22(3):307–16.

7. Richards TB, Henley SJ, Puckett MC, et al. Lung cancer survival in the United States by race and stage (2001-2009): findings from the CONCORD-2 study. Cancer 2017;123(Suppl 24):5079–99.

8. Dalwadi SM, Lewis GD, Bernicker EH, et al. Disparities in the treatment and outcome of stage I non-small-cell lung cancer in the 21st Century. Clin Lung Cancer 2019;20(3):194–200.

9. Wolf A, Alpert N, Tran BV, et al. Persistence of racial disparities in early-stage lung cancer treatment. J Thorac Cardiovasc Surg 2019;157(4):1670–9.e4.

10. Williams CD, Alpert N, Redding TS, et al. Racial differences in treatment and survival among veterans and non-veterans with stage I NSCLC: an evaluation of Veterans Affairs and SEER-Medicare populations. Cancer Epidemiol Biomark Prev 2020;29(1):112–8.

11. Xu L, Zhang G, Song S, et al. Surgery for small cell lung cancer: a Surveillance, Epidemiology, and End Results (SEER) survey from 2010 to 2015. Medicine (Baltimore) 2019;98(40):e17214.

12. Mulligan CR, Meram AD, Proctor CD, et al. Unlimited access to care: effect on racial disparity and prognostic factors in lung cancer. Cancer Epidemiol Biomark Prev 2006;15(1):25–31.

13. Vyfhuis MAL, Bhooshan N, Moliṭoris J, et al. Clinical outcomes of black vs. non-black patients with locally advanced non-small cell lung cancer. Lung Cancer 2017;114:44–9.

14. Merritt RE, Abdel-Rasoul M, D'Souza DM, et al. Racial disparities in overall survival and surgical treatment for early stage lung cancer by facility type. Clin Lung Cancer 2021. https://doi.org/10.1016/j.cllc.2021.01.007.

15. Bryant AS, Cerfolio RJ. Impact of race on outcomes of patients with non-small cell lung cancer. J Thorac Oncol 2008;3(7):711–5.

16. Check DK, Albers KB, Uppal KM, et al. Examining the role of access to care: racial/ethnic differences in receipt of resection for early-stage non-small cell lung cancer among integrated system members and non-members. Lung Cancer Amst Neth 2018;125:51–6.

17. Shugarman LR, Mack K, Sorbero MES, et al. Race and sex differences in the receipt of timely and appropriate lung cancer treatment. Med Care 2009;47(7):774–81.

18. Rapp JL, Tuminello S, Alpert N, et al. Disparities in surgical recommendation for stage I non-small cell lung cancer. Am J Clin Oncol 2020;43(10):741–7.

19. Esnaola NF, Gebregziabher M, Knott K, et al. Underuse of surgical resection for localized, non-small cell lung cancer among whites and African Americans in South Carolina. Ann Thorac Surg 2008;86(1):220–6 [discussion 227].

20. Steele CB, Pisu M, Richardson LC. Urban/rural patterns in receipt of treatment for non-small cell lung cancer among black and white Medicare beneficiaries, 2000-2003. J Natl Med Assoc 2011;103(8):711–8.

21. Farjah F, Wood DE, Yanez ND, et al. Racial disparities among patients with lung cancer who were recommended operative therapy. Arch Surg 2009;144(1):14–8.

22. Corso CD, Park HS, Kim AW, et al. Racial disparities in the use of SBRT for treating early-stage lung cancer. Lung Cancer 2015;89(2):133–8.

23. Ezer N, Mhango G, Bagiella E, et al. Racial disparities in resection of early stage non-small cell lung cancer: variability among surgeons. Med Care 2020;58(4):392–8.

24. LaPar DJ, Bhamidipati CM, Harris DA, et al. Gender, race, and socioeconomic status affects outcomes after lung cancer resections in the United States. Ann Thorac Surg 2011;92(2):434–9.

25. Mehta RS, Lenzner D, Argiris A. Race and health disparities in patient refusal of surgery for early-stage non-small cell lung cancer: a SEER cohort study. Ann Surg Oncol 2012;19(3):722–7.

26. Lin JJ, Mhango G, Wall MM, et al. Cultural factors associated with racial disparities in lung cancer care. Ann Am Thorac Soc 2014;11(4):489–95.

27. Cykert S, Eng E, Walker P, et al. A system-based intervention to reduce black-white disparities in the treatment of early stage lung cancer: a pragmatic trial at five cancer centers. Cancer Med 2019;8(3):1095–102.

28. Williams CD, Salama JK, Moghanaki D, et al. Impact of race on treatment and survival among U.S. veterans with early-stage lung cancer. J Thorac Oncol 2016;11(10):1672–81.

29. Blackstock AW, Herndon JE, Paskett ED, et al. Similar outcomes between African American and non-African American patients with extensive-stage small-cell lung carcinoma: report from the Cancer and Leukemia Group B. J Clin Oncol 2006;24(3):407–12.

30. Jones CC, Mercaldo SF, Blume JD, et al. Racial disparities in lung cancer survival: the contribution of

stage, treatment, and ancestry. J Thorac Oncol 2018;13(10):1464–73.

31. Klugman M, Xue X, Hosgood HD. Race/ethnicity and lung cancer survival in the United States: a meta-analysis. Cancer Causes Control 2019; 30(11):1231–41.

32. Klugman M, Xue X, Ginsberg M, et al. Hispanics/ Latinos in the Bronx have improved survival in non-small cell lung cancer compared with non-Hispanic whites. J Racial Ethn Health Disparities 2020;7(2): 316–26.

33. Smith CB, Bonomi M, Packer S, et al. Disparities in lung cancer stage, treatment and survival among American Indians and Alaskan Natives. Lung Cancer 2011;72(2):160–4.

34. Fesinmeyer MD, Goulart B, Blough DK, et al. Lung cancer histology, stage, treatment, and survival in American Indians and Alaska Natives and whites. Cancer 2010;116(20):4810–6.

35. Chang ET, Shema SJ, Wakelee HA, et al. Uncovering disparities in survival after non-small-cell lung cancer among Asian/Pacific Islander ethnic populations in California. Cancer Epidemiol Biomark Prev 2009; 18(8):2248–55.

36. Subramanian J, Govindan R. Lung cancer in never smokers: a review. J Clin Oncol 2007;25(5):561–70.

37. Jemal A, Miller KD, Ma J, et al. Higher lung cancer incidence in young women than young men in the United States. N Engl J Med 2018;378(21): 1999–2009.

38. Titan AL, He H, Lui N, et al. The influence of hormone replacement therapy on lung cancer incidence and mortality. J Thorac Cardiovasc Surg 2020;159(4): 1546–56.e4.

39. Elkbuli A, Byrne MM, Zhao W, et al. Gender disparities in lung cancer survival from an enriched Florida population-based cancer registry. Ann Med Surg 2020;60:680–5.

40. Wisnivesky JP, Halm EA. Sex differences in lung cancer survival: do tumors behave differently in elderly women? J Clin Oncol 2007;25(13):1705–12.

41. Cerfolio RJ, Bryant AS, Scott E, et al. Women with pathologic stage I, II, and III non-small cell lung cancer have better survival than men. Chest 2006; 130(6):1796–802.

42. Tong BC, Kosinski AS, Burfeind WR, et al. Sex differences in early outcomes after lung cancer resection: analysis of the Society of Thoracic Surgeons General Thoracic Database. J Thorac Cardiovasc Surg 2014;148(1):13–8.

43. Brahmer JR, Dahlberg SE, Gray RJ, et al. Sex differences in outcome with bevacizumab therapy: analysis of patients with advanced-stage non-small cell lung cancer treated with or without bevacizumab in combination with paclitaxel and carboplatin in the Eastern Cooperative Oncology Group Trial 4599. J Thorac Oncol 2011;6(1):103–8.

44. Rivera MP. Lung cancer in women: differences in epidemiology, biology, histology, and treatment outcomes. Semin Respir Crit Care Med 2013;34(6): 792–801.

45. Institute of Medicine (US) Board on the Health of Select Populations. Collecting sexual orientation and gender identity data in electronic health records: workshop summary. National Academies Press (US); 2013. Available at: http://www.ncbi. nlm.nih.gov/books/NBK132859/. Accessed May 19, 2021.

46. Nadpara PA, Madhavan SS, Tworek C, et al. Guideline-concordant lung cancer care and associated health outcomes among elderly patients in the United States. J Geriatr Oncol 2015;6(2):101–10.

47. Cassidy RJ, Zhang X, Switchenko JM, et al. Health care disparities among octogenarians and nonagenarians with stage III lung cancer. Cancer 2018; 124(4):775–84.

48. Caprario LC, Kent DM, Strauss GM. Effects of chemotherapy on survival of elderly patients with small-cell lung cancer: analysis of the SEER-Medicare database. J Thorac Oncol 2013;8(10): 1272–81.

49. Thomas A, Chen Y, Yu T, et al. Trends and characteristics of young non-small cell lung cancer patients in the United States. Front Oncol 2015;5:113.

50. Iezzoni LI, Ngo LH, Li D, et al. Treatment disparities for disabled Medicare beneficiaries with stage I non-small cell lung cancer. Arch Phys Med Rehabil 2008; 89(4):595–601.

51. Schwartz KL, Crossley-May H, Vigneau FD, et al. Race, socioeconomic status and stage at diagnosis for five common malignancies. Cancer Causes Control 2003;14(8):761–6.

52. Halpern MT, Ward EM, Pavluck AL, et al. Association of insurance status and ethnicity with cancer stage at diagnosis for 12 cancer sites: a retrospective analysis. Lancet Oncol 2008;9(3):222–31.

53. Ward EM, Fedewa SA, Cokkinides V, et al. The association of insurance and stage at diagnosis among patients aged 55 to 74 years in the National Cancer Database. Cancer J Sudbury Mass 2010;16(6): 614–21.

54. Slatore CG, Au DH, Gould MK, American Thoracic Society Disparities in Healthcare Group. An official American Thoracic Society systematic review: insurance status and disparities in lung cancer practices and outcomes. Am J Respir Crit Care Med 2010; 182(9):1195–205.

55. Yang R, Cheung MC, Byrne MM, et al. Do racial or socioeconomic disparities exist in lung cancer treatment? Cancer 2010;116(10):2437–47.

56. Ebner PJ, Ding L, Kim AW, et al. The effect of socioeconomic status on treatment and mortality in non-small cell lung cancer patients. Ann Thorac Surg 2020;109(1):225–32.

57. Jiang X, Lin G, Islam KMM. Socioeconomic factors related to surgical treatment for localized, non-small cell lung cancer. Soc Sci Med 2017;175:52–7.

58. Ou S-HI, Zell JA, Ziogas A, et al. Low socioeconomic status is a poor prognostic factor for survival in stage I nonsmall cell lung cancer and is independent of surgical treatment, race, and marital status. Cancer 2008;112(9):2011–20.

59. Toubat O, Atay SM, Kim AW, et al. Disparities in guideline-concordant treatment for pathologic N1 non-small cell lung cancer. Ann Thorac Surg 2020; 109(5):1512–20.

60. Duma N, Idossa DW, Durani U, et al. Influence of sociodemographic factors on treatment decisions in non-small-cell lung cancer. Clin Lung Cancer 2020; 21(3):e115–29.

61. Khullar OV, Gillespie T, Nickleach DC, et al. Socioeconomic risk factors for long-term mortality after pulmonary resection for lung cancer: an analysis of more than 90,000 patients from the National Cancer Data Base. J Am Coll Surg 2015;220(2):156–68.e4.

62. Melvan JN, Sancheti MS, Gillespie T, et al. Nonclinical factors associated with 30-day mortality after lung cancer resection: an analysis of 215,000 patients using the National Cancer Data base. J Am Coll Surg 2015;221(2):550–63.

63. Zhou K, Shi H, Chen R, et al. Association of race, socioeconomic factors, and treatment characteristics with overall survival in patients with limited-stage small cell lung cancer. JAMA Netw Open 2021; 4(1):e2032276.

64. Herndon JE, Kornblith AB, Holland JC, et al. Patient education level as a predictor of survival in lung cancer clinical trials. J Clin Oncol 2008;26(25):4116–23.

65. Johnson AM, Hines RB, Johnson JA, et al. Treatment and survival disparities in lung cancer: the effect of social environment and place of residence. Lung Cancer 2014;83(3):401–7.

66. Shugarman LR, Sorbero MES, Tian H, et al. An exploration of urban and rural differences in lung cancer survival among Medicare beneficiaries. Am J Public Health 2008;98(7):1280–7.

67. Atkins GT, Kim T, Munson J. Residence in rural areas of the United States and lung cancer mortality. Disease incidence, treatment disparities, and stage-specific survival. Ann Am Thorac Soc 2017;14(3): 403–11.

68. Nicoli CD, Sprague BL, Anker CJ, et al. Association of rurality with survival and guidelines-concordant management in early-stage non-small cell lung cancer. Am J Clin Oncol 2019;42(7):607–14.

69. Ray MA, Faris NR, Derrick A, et al. Rurality, stage-stratified use of treatment modalities, and survival of non-small cell lung cancer. Chest 2020;158(2): 787–96.

70. Backhus LM, Hayanga AJ, Au D, et al. The effect of provider density on lung cancer survival among blacks and whites in the United States. J Thorac Oncol 2013;8(5):549–53.

71. Hayanga AJ, Zeliadt SB, Backhus LM. Residential segregation and lung cancer mortality in the United States. JAMA Surg 2013;148(1):37–42.

Social Disparities in Benign Lung Diseases

Jairo Espinosa, MD[a],*, Siva Raja, MD, PhD, FACS[b]

KEYWORDS

- Social disparities in benign lung diseases • COVID-19 • Tuberculosis • COPD • Asthma
- Sarcoidosis • Cystic fibrosis • Idiopathic pulmonary fibrosis

KEY POINTS

- Socioeconomic disparities in benign lung diseases are a global issue that were most recently highlighted by the COVID-19 pandemic, but also include other infectious global diseases such as tuberculosis and fungal diseases.
- Socioeconomic disparities in obstructive lung disease have been identified since the 1980's and include disparities amongst neighborhoods, races, and health literacy.
- Socioeconomic disparities in restrictive lung disease are seen in cystic fibrosis, idiopathic pulmonary fibrosis, and cystic fibrosis are present amongst lower socioeconomic status patients and extends to the point of which patient will get a transplant or not.

INTRODUCTION

Socioeconomic disparities impact all health care, including benign lung diseases. Disparities in benign lung diseases came to the forefront of global health with the COVID-19 pandemic. In this chapter, we will be reviewing the socioeconomic disparities in benign lung disease from both a United States perspective as well as a global perspective. We will cover the spectrum of infectious, obstructive, and restrictive lung disease and review the evidence on how social disparities affect these populations and their access to medical care.

SOCIOECONOMIC DISPARITIES IN INFECTIOUS LUNG DISEASE
COVID-19

COVID-19 has garnered more attention and research in recent times than any other pulmonic infection. To date, the viral infection has caused over 3 million deaths worldwide, with over half a million deaths in the United States alone.[1] SARS-CoV-2 (severe acute respiratory syndrome-coronavirus) the virus that causes COVID-19

(coronavirus disease of 2019) is a coronavirus in the order of Nidovirales in the family of coronaviridae that was first discovered in December 2019 in Wuhan, China.[2] SARS-CoV-2 is an enveloped single-stranded RNA virus that uses its receptor-binding domain in the spike protein on its envelope to bind to the ACE2 receptor in human cells and infect them.[2] Shortly after its discovery, the United States of America became the epicenter of the pandemic. This event quickly exposed the racial and socioeconomic disparities that exist in our society. COVID-19 infection data have highlighted, more clearly than ever, the racial, ethnic, urban, and intercounty/city socioeconomic disparities deeply enrooted within health care.

COVID-19 infections in the United States of America has occurred at a much higher rate in the Hispanic and black populations than in the white population.[3] The rate of COVID-19 infections in the United States as of July 2020 was markedly higher in the Latino and Black populations, at 73 cases per 100,000 and 62 cases per 100,000 respectively, when compared with the white population at 23 cases per 100,000 in the white population.[3] Similar trends can be seen in the COVID-19

[a] Department of Thoracic Surgery, Temple University Hospital, 3401 N. Broad Street, Suite C501, Parkinson Pavilion, Philadelphia, PA 19140, USA; [b] Department of Thoracic Surgery, Cleveland Clinic 9500 Euclid Avenue, Cleveland, Ohio 44195, USA
* Corresponding author.
E-mail address: Jairo.espinosa@tuhs.temple.edu

Thorac Surg Clin 32 (2022) 43–49
https://doi.org/10.1016/j.thorsurg.2021.09.006

thoracic.theclinics.com

mortality data from New York City and Chicago. The combined Hispanic and black resident COVID-19 mortality accounted for 58.6% and 75.5% of the COVID-19 deaths, respectively, in NYC and Chicago despite making up only 53.4% and 58.4% of the population in those 2 cities.[3–6] As many have suggested (especially early in the pandemic's course), that rates of infection are affected by testing availability, Credit and colleagues evaluated the neighborhood level COVID-19 infection data for these 2 large metropolitan areas. In the study, the authors studied neighborhoods in Chicago and New York City based on majority race per neighborhood, socioeconomic status based on income, variables affecting "healthy" living environments, testing availability, and positive testing rate.[3] Yet, despite the non-Hispanic white neighborhoods having a significantly higher accessibility to COVID-19 testing, the predominantly non-Hispanic black and Hispanic neighborhoods had a significantly higher amount of COVID-19 cases.[3]

Similar trends in COVID-19 mortality with racial disparities, socioeconomic disparities are quite striking when comparing urban to rural America. In a national review of county-level data, Paul and colleagues reviewed data from over 3100 counties across 48 states regarding COVID-19 infections and deaths; as well as socioeconomic factors including but not limited to education level, rural versus urban designation, and racial/ethnicity data.[7] In this study, the authors found that the COVID-19 mortality rate was significantly higher in the urban population than in the rural population— 65 per 100,000 versus 50 per 100,000, respectively.[7] Furthermore, the interplay between regional variability and rare is very enlightening. When evaluating the urban county data, the authors found that despite the mortality rate being significantly lower in the rural population, when comparing whites and blacks, the COVID-19 mortality rates increased by 3.4% for every 5% in residential segregation, and mortality increased by 47.9% for every 5% in unemployment rate.[7] This study is significant because it highlights how residential segregation negatively impacts the black population even when mortality seems to be lower in a particular region/county. Also, unfortunately, the unemployment and income inequities are not unexpected findings, given that the United States ranked 30 out of 32 in developed countries for income-based health inequalities.[8]

Tuberculosis

A pulmonary infection that has plagued mankind for many millennia is tuberculosis. Advances in medical therapy had largely mitigated its lethality until the resurgence of multidrug-resistant variants. Despite the incidence of tuberculosis being very low in the overall population in the modern era (3.2 per 100,000, and the lowest it has been since 1953), it still continues to affect vulnerable populations such as inmates as well as disadvantaged groups such as minorities, and lower socioeconomic populations at a disproportionately higher rate.[9–12] Studies have shown that inmates at the state and federal level have a 4 to 5 times higher incidence of tuberculosis than the nonincarcerated population.[11] Also, despite the fact that these individuals are incarcerated and should have the easiest access to follow-up and compliance—inmates are much less likely to complete treatment when compared with the nonincarcerated population, 76.8% versus 89.4% completion rate, respectively.[11] In another study of tuberculosis rates in the United States based on socioeconomic status, Olson and colleagues found that patients in the lower quartile of socioeconomic status had 4.8 to 7.2 times higher TB rates than those in the highest quartile.[13]

Fungal Infection

Finally, fungal pulmonary infections which are ubiquitous and regional are not immune to socioeconomic disparities. One example of this is blastomycosis. Blastomycosis is a pulmonic/systemic infection caused by *Blastomyces dermatitidis* that is transmitted via airborne and is found in states near the Ohio River Valley, Mississippi River, and Great Lakes.[14,15] In a recent review by Sorvillo and colleagues, blacks and Native Americans were significantly more likely to die from blastomycosis than whites.[15]

SOCIOECONOMIC DISPARITIES IN OBSTRUCTIVE LUNG DISEASE

Socioeconomic disparities in obstructive lung disease are a heavily researched field with disparities in asthma patients being known since the 1980s.[16] This is very significant given that asthma is the most common noncommunicable disease in children that affects 339 million people worldwide and has an annual health care cost of around $56 billion in the United States alone.[17,18] Socioeconomic disparities in asthma have been found to not only be a major issue in the United States, but also at the international level. In the United States, African-American children with asthma have 2 to 3 times higher rates of emergency room visits and hospital admissions and 4.9 times higher asthma mortality rate when compared with non-Hispanic white children.[16,19,20] Hispanic children with asthma are also at an increased risk with 2 times higher rates of emergency room visits and hospital admissions and 1.5 times higher asthma mortality rate when compared with non-Hispanic white children.[19]

Asthma

As mentioned, socioeconomic disparities are unfortunately a global issue. Asthma has been found to have a higher prevalence in lower socioeconomic groups when categorized based on education or social class in North America, Europe, and Australia.[21] Previous risk factors that have been explored to explain these disparities include smoking, body mass index, sex, age, occupational exposures, atopy, childhood infections, domestic mold growth, and family size. All these risk factors were included in a multi-continent cross-sectional study including 32 centers using data from the European Community Respiratory Health Survey (ECRHS) and the higher prevalence in the lower socioeconomic groups continued to be significant.[21]

Air pollution exposure is another significant risk factor that may explain the socioeconomic disparities found in asthma. Multiple studies have found that air pollution exposure at an early age and/or during pregnancy increases the risk of childhood asthma.[22–24] Early-life exposure to nitrogen dioxide and fine particulate matter (both markers of pollution) has been found to increase the risk of developing childhood asthma.[25] When comparing children with high concentration versus low concentration early life exposure to nitrogen dioxide or fine particulate matter; the high concentration exposure children have 1.25 times higher odds of developing childhood asthma.[25] Unfortunately, there is a positive correlation/association in children living in high poverty neighborhoods to both nitrogen dioxide and fine particulate matter exposure and thus lower socioeconomic status children are at an increased risk of developing childhood asthma.[25]

A more recent, interesting finding in asthma patients is the association of vitamin D deficiency and asthma exacerbations. This is a significant finding given that adults and children of lower socioeconomic status tend to have higher rates of vitamin deficiencies and malnutrition.[26] Children with mild to moderate persistent asthma and vitamin D deficiency are at an increased risk of asthma-related emergency room visits and hospitalizations; even after adjusting for age, sex, BMI, and asthma severity.[27] Specifically for vitamin D, African-American adolescents are 20 times more likely to be vitamin D deficient than non-Hispanic white adolescents.[20] Also, in Costa Rican children with asthma; lower vitamin D levels have been found to be inversely related to asthma severity and for every log (10) unit increase in vitamin D levels there is a decrease in hospitalizations, use of antiinflammatory medications, and increased airway responsiveness.[28]

Another "explanation" that has been proposed to explain the socioeconomic disparities seen when comparing the African American, non-Hispanic white, and Hispanic populations with asthma is the concept of *health literacy*. *Health literacy* is defined as, "the degree to which individuals have the capacity to obtain, process, and understand basic health information and services needed to make appropriate health decisions."[29] Although multiple studies have found that taking into account health literacy "significantly reduces" health disparities, others have found that although limited health literacy could partially explain some of the racial disparities in emergency room visits in asthma patients, the hospitalization rates could not be explained based on health literacy alone.[30–36] Yet, this terminology must be used with caution as a way to dismiss socioeconomic health disparities. As to say that Hispanics and African American individuals are less literate and thus less capable of making appropriate health decision seems in itself to be a disparity secondary to the educational opportunities and financial limitations that these individuals face when compared with non-Hispanic individuals.

Chronic Obstructive Pulmonary Disease

Chronic obstructive pulmonary disease (COPD) is another common obstructive lung disease with significant socioeconomic disparities. Socioeconomic status has been found to have an inverse relationship with COPD. COPD patients with lower socioeconomic status have been found to be twice as likely to have worse outcomes as those with higher socioeconomic status.[37] Living in a socioeconomic disadvantaged neighborhood or a "poor" neighborhood can be bad for one's health. The effect of living in a poor neighborhood has been shown to have a negative effect on COPD and other chronic conditions; with individuals living in poor neighborhoods tending to have worse outcomes than those living in less disadvantaged neighborhoods.[38–40] Interestingly enough, it has also been found that moving from a poor neighborhood to a less disadvantaged neighborhood can have positive health effects.[41,42] In COPD, patients residing in the most disadvantaged neighborhoods have been found to have a 56% higher rate of COPD exacerbations, 98% higher rate of severe COPD exacerbations, and 24.6 m less 6-minute walk distance when compared with individuals living in the least disadvantaged neighborhoods.[40] This finding was recently further studied by using SPIROMICS (subpopulations and intermediate outcome measures in COPD Study) data as well as United States census data to further evaluate COPD outcomes in African Americans when compared with non-Hispanic white Americans.[43] It was found that black individuals have worse COPD symptoms and worse quality of life when compared with white individuals. Some of these findings may be explained based on individual socioeconomic status and neighborhood disparity/poverty.[43] However, even when taking into account individual socioeconomic status and neighborhood disparity black individuals continue to have 1.71 times higher rate of severe COPD exacerbations and worse CT (computed tomography) findings.[43]

SOCIOECONOMIC DISPARITIES IN RESTRICTIVE LUNG DISEASE
Sarcoidosis

Sarcoidosis is a multisystem autoimmune granulomatous disease that can affect any organ in your body, but typically affects your lungs, skin, and lymph nodes.[44,45] Sarcoidosis is more commonly seen in females than males and in the United States of America, the race most commonly affected is African Americans.[45] Its pulmonary involvement is characterized by symmetric hilar lymphadenopathy seen in chests X-ray and restrictive lung disease.[46] Pathologically it is characterized by nonnecrotizing granulomas.[46] Unfortunately, low-income patients, African American patients, and less educated patients have been found to have more severe disease at presentation.[47–49] Low-income patients have been found to have significantly higher sarcoidosis-related comorbidities, steroid-related comorbidities, lower quality of life, and be further impacted financially secondary to sarcoidosis with up to 46% of sarcoidosis patients being severely financially affected by the disease and 31% of the cohort having to quit their job.[47]

Idiopathic Pulmonary Fibrosis

Another restrictive lung disease with socioeconomic disparities is idiopathic pulmonary fibrosis. Unfortunately, the disparities in this disease are not as well studied. Idiopathic pulmonary fibrosis is a progressive, chronic interstitial, restrictive lung disease without a cure.[50] In a nationwide inpatient database review of 148,000 adults hospitalized in the United States with idiopathic pulmonary fibrosis patients with Medicaid, no insurance,

and lower socioeconomic status were less likely to receive a lung transplant.[50] Also, they found that those with Medicaid and uninsured were less likely to undergo a lung biopsy or be discharged to a rehabilitation facility.[50] As mentioned by the authors—these findings are similar to those seen in cystic fibrosis patients and in Hispanic patients on liver transplant lists.[51,52] Further highlighting the need for health care reform in the United States of America. In addition, Hispanic and black minorities with idiopathic pulmonary fibrosis have been found to be less likely to get listed for lung transplantation when compared with non-Hispanic white and Asian patients. When these Hispanic and black populations with idiopathic pulmonary fibrosis are listed for lung transplantation, they have more than 4 times increased risk of death whereas awaiting transplantation when compared with non-Hispanic white and Asian patients even when taking into account age, gender, spirometry, transplantation status, and smoking history.[53]

SOCIOECONOMIC DISPARITIES IN CYSTIC FIBROSIS

Cystic fibrosis is a common autosomal recessive disease that most commonly affects Caucasian individuals.[54] The disease is caused by mutations in the cystic fibrosis transmembrane conductance regulator (CFTR) channel which leads to abnormal secretions throughout the body.[55] Cystic fibrosis heavily affects the lungs with respiratory infections being the most common cause of death in this patient population.[56] Gender disparities in cystic fibrosis are a well-known and studied phenomenon that has been acknowledged since the 1990s.[56,57] Multiple studies have shown that women with cystic fibrosis have a shorter life expectancy than men with cystic fibrosis and that they tend to acquire pseudomonas aeruginosa infection at an earlier age than men; leading to a faster decline in lung function and thus shorter lifespan.[56,58,59] Harness-Brumley and colleagues, also found through a large retrospective cohort analysis of over 32,000 patients that women with cystic fibrosis acquire a variety of gram positive, gram negative, fungal, and mycobacterial infections before men with many of these infections occurring as early as before puberty and leading to a decreased lifespan.[56]

Tobacco smoke exposure has also been found to be detrimental in patients with cystic fibrosis. Children who have been exposed to tobacco smoke are found to have an FEV1 4.7% lower than children with cystic fibrosis and no tobacco smoke exposure.[55] The effect of smoke exposure on FEV1 has been found to be greater in socioeconomic disadvantaged children when compared with the less disadvantaged (3.2% vs 1.2%).[55] Interestingly enough, for every $10,000 increase in household income—the median FEV1 in children increases by 0.2%—highlighting the significant socioeconomic disparities when comparing the poor, to the rich.[55]

SUMMARY

Benign lung diseases are subject to the same social disparities as many other maladies. Nevertheless, these diseases highlight the interconnected nature of social, economic, and racial disparities as it pertains to the prevalence of lung disease as well as the delivery and access to health care in the modern era. To acknowledge this disparity and its root causes are the first steps in creating durable change. The next steps involve systemic changes to our health care system to improve access to medicine, both preventive and therapeutic. Although we can debate whether health care is a right or a privilege, no one disagrees that access to health care is a necessity. It is one that we need to resolve in our time and not pass the burden to the future. Specifically, we as thoracic surgeons must educate ourselves on the impact of social disparity on disease processes, vulnerable population, and the care that we deliver.

CLINICS CARE POINTS

- SARS-CoV-2 the virus that causes COVID-19 has highlighted the racial, ethnic, urban, and inter-county/city socioeconomic disparities deeply enrooted within healthcare and the need for improvement to diminish these inequalities.

- Women with cystic fibrosis have a shorter life expectancy than men with cystic fibrosis and they tend to acquire pseudomonas aeruginosa infection at an earlier age leading to a faster decline in lung function and thus shorter lifespan.

- Hispanic and black patients with idiopathic pulmonary fibrosis listed for lung transplantation have more than 4 times increased risk of death while awaiting transplantation when compared to non-Hispanic white and Asian patients.

- COPD patients residing in disadvantaged neighborhoods have been found to have higher rate of COPD exacerbations, higher rate of severe COPD exacerbations, and less six minute walk distance when compared to individuals living in the least disadvantaged neighborhoods.

REFERENCES

1. Coronavirus world map: tracking the global outbreak - The New York Times. Available at: https://www.nytimes.com/interactive/2020/world/coronavirus-maps.html. Accessed April 21, 2021.

2. Mohamadian M, Chiti H, Shoghli A, et al. COVID-19: virology, biology and novel laboratory diagnosis. J Gene Med 2021;23(2):1–11. https://doi.org/10.1002/jgm.3303.

3. Credit K. Neighbourhood inequity: exploring the factors underlying racial and ethnic disparities in COVID-19 testing and infection rates using ZIP code data in Chicago and New York. Reg Sci Policy Pract 2020;12(6):1249–71.

4. COVID-19 statistics | IDPH. Available at: http://www.dph.illinois.gov/COVID19/COVID19-statistics. Accessed April 21, 2021.

5. U.S. Census bureau QuickFacts: New York city, New York. Available at: https://www.census.gov/quickfacts/newyorkcitynewyork. Accessed April 21, 2021.

6. U.S. Census Bureau QuickFacts: Chicago city, Illinois. https://www.census.gov/quickfacts/chicagocityillinois. Accessed April 21, 2021.

7. Paul R, Arif A, Pokhrel K, et al. The association of social determinants of health with COVID-19 mortality in rural and urban counties. J Rural Heal 2021;37(2):278–86. https://doi.org/10.1111/jrh.12557.

8. Hero JO, Zaslavsky AM, Blendon RJ. The United States leads other nations in differences by income in perceptions of health and health care. Health Aff 2017;36(6):1032–40. https://doi.org/10.1377/hlthaff.2017.0006.

9. Trends in tuberculosis — United States. Available at: https://www.cdc.gov/mmwr/preview/mmwrhtml/mm6311a2.htm. Accessed April 23, 2021.

10. Schneider E, Moore M, Castro KG. Epidemiology of tuberculosis in the United States. Clin Chest Med 2005;26(2):183–95. https://doi.org/10.1016/j.ccm.2005.02.007.

11. MacNeil JR, Lobato MN, Moore M. An unanswered health disparity: tuberculosis among correctional inmates, 1993 through 2003. Am J Public Health 2005;95(10):1800–5.

12. Noppert GA, Wilson ML, Clarke P, et al. Race and nativity are major determinants of tuberculosis in the U.S.: evidence of health disparities in tuberculosis incidence in Michigan, 2004-2012. BMC Public Health 2017;17(1):1–11. https://doi.org/10.1186/s12889-017-4461-y.

13. Olson NA, Davidow AL, Winston CA, et al. A national study of socioeconomic status and tuberculosis rates by country of birth, United States, 1996-2005. BMC Public Health 2012;12(1):1. https://doi.org/10.1186/1471-2458-12-365.

14. Hospenthal DR, Rinaldi MG. Diagnosis and treatment of human Mycoses. Totowa, NJ: Humana Press; 2008.

15. Khuu D, Shafir S, Bristow B, et al. Blastomycosis mortality rates, United States, 1990-2010. Emerg Infect Dis 2014;20(11):1789–94. https://doi.org/10.3201/eid2011.131175.

16. Volerman A, Chin MH, Press VG. Solutions for asthma disparities. Pediatrics 2017;139(3). https://doi.org/10.1542/peds.2016-2546.

17. Asthma. Available at: https://www.who.int/en/newsroom/fact-sheets/detail/asthma. Accessed April 25, 2021.

18. Barnett SBL, Nurmagambetov TA. Costs of asthma in the United States: 2002-2007. J Allergy Clin Immunol 2011;127(1):145–52. https://doi.org/10.1016/j.jaci.2010.10.020.

19. National surveillance of asthma: United States, 2001-2010 - PubMed. Available at: https://pubmed.ncbi.nlm.nih.gov/24252609/. Accessed April 25, 2021.

20. Saintonge S, Bang H, Gerber LM. Implications of a new definition of vitamin D deficiency in a multiracial US adolescent population: the national health and nutrition examination survey III. Pediatrics 2009;123(3): 797–803. https://doi.org/10.1542/peds.2008-1195.

21. Basagaña X, Sunyer J, Kogevinas M, et al. Socioeconomic status and asthma prevalence in young adults: The European community respiratory health survey. Am J Epidemiol 2004;160(2):178–88. https://doi.org/10.1093/aje/kwh186.

22. Pennington AF, Strickland MJ, Klein M, et al. Measurement error in mobile source air pollution exposure estimates due to residential mobility during pregnancy. J Expo Sci Environ Epidemiol 2017; 27(5):513–20. https://doi.org/10.1038/jes.2016.66.

23. Nishimura KK, Galanter JM, Roth LA, et al. Early-Life air pollution and asthma risk in minority children the GALA II and SAGE II studies. Am J Respir Crit Care Med 2013;188(3):309–18. https://doi.org/10.1164/rccm.201302-0264OC.

24. Hsu HHL, Chiu YHM, Coull BA, et al. Prenatal particulate air pollution and asthma onset in urban children: Identifying sensitive windows and sex differences. Am J Respir Crit Care Med 2015; 192(9):1052–9. https://doi.org/10.1164/rccm.201504-0658OC.

25. Kravitz-Wirtz N, Teixeira S, Hajat A, et al. Early-life air pollution exposure, neighborhood poverty, and childhood asthma in the United States, 1990–2014. Int J Environ Res Public Health 2018;15(6):1–14. https://doi.org/10.3390/ijerph15061114.

26. Hill TD, Graham LM, Divgi V. Racial disparities in pediatric asthma: a review of the literature. Curr Allergy Asthma Rep 2011;11(1):85–90. https://doi.org/10.1007/s11882-010-0159-2.

27. Brehm JM, Schuemann B, Fuhlbrigge AL, et al. Serum vitamin D levels and severe asthma exacerbations in the Childhood Asthma Management Program study. J Allergy Clin Immunol 2010; 126(1):52–8.e5. https://doi.org/10.1016/j.jaci.2010.03.043.

28. Brehm JM, Celedón JC, Soto-Quiros ME, et al. Serum vitamin D levels and markers of severity of childhood asthma in Costa Rica. Am J Respir Crit Care Med 2009;179(9):765–71.

29. Nielsen-Bohlman L. Health literacy a prescription to end confusion. In: Nielsen-Bohlman L, Panzer AM, Kindig DA, editors. Washington, DC: National Academies Press; 2004. https://doi.org/10.17226/10883.

30. Curtis LM, Wolf MS, Weiss KB, et al. The impact of health literacy and socioeconomic status on asthma disparities. J Asthma 2012;49(2):178–83. https://doi.org/10.3109/02770903.2011.648297.

31. Bennett CL, Ferreira MR, Davis TC, et al. Relation between literacy, race, and stage of presentation among low- income patients with prostate cancer. J Clin Oncol 1998;16(9):3101–4. https://doi.org/10.1200/JCO.1998.16.9.3101.

32. Howard DH, Sentell T, Gazmararian JA. Impact of health literacy on socioeconomic and racial differences in health in an elderly population. J Gen Intern Med 2006;21(8):857–61. https://doi.org/10.1111/j.1525-1497.2006.00530.x.

33. Sentell TL, Halpin HA. Importance of adult literacy in understanding health disparities. J Gen Intern Med 2006;21(8):862–6. https://doi.org/10.1111/j.1525-1497.2006.00538.x.

34. Wolf MS, Knight SJ, Lyons EA, et al. Literacy, race, and PSA level among low-income men newly diagnosed with prostate cancer. Urology 2006;68(1):89–93. https://doi.org/10.1016/j.urology.2006.01.064.

35. Osborn CY, Paasche-Orlow MK, Davis TC, et al. Health literacy. An overlooked factor in understanding HIV health disparities. Am J Prev Med 2007;33(5):374–8. https://doi.org/10.1016/j.amepre.2007.07.022.

36. Bennett IM, Chen J, Soroui JS, et al. The contribution of health literacy to disparities in self-rated health status and preventive health behaviors in older adults. Ann Fam Med 2009;7(3):204–11. https://doi.org/10.1370/afm.940.

37. Gershon AS, Dolmage TE, Stephenson A, et al. Chronic obstructive pulmonary disease and socioeconomic status: a systematic review. COPD 2012; 9(3):216–26. https://doi.org/10.3109/15412555.2011.648030.

38. Acevedo-Garcia D, Osypuk TL, McArdle N, et al. Toward a policy-relevant analysis of geographic and racial/ethnic disparities in child health. Health Aff 2008;27(2):321–33. https://doi.org/10.1377/hlthaff.27.2.321.

39. Ludwig J, Duncan GJ, Gennetian LA, et al. Neighborhood effects on the long-term well-being of low-income adults. Science 2012;337(6101):1505–10. https://doi.org/10.1126/science.1224648.

40. Galiatsatos P, Woo H, Paulin LM, et al. The association between neighborhood socioeconomic disadvantage and chronic obstructive pulmonary disease. Int J Chron Obstruct Pulmon Dis 2020;15: 981–93. https://doi.org/10.2147/COPD.S238933.

41. Sciandra M, Sanbonmatsu L, Duncan GJ, et al. Long-term effects of the moving to opportunity residential mobility experiment on crime and delinquency. J Exp Criminol 2013;9(4):451–89. https://doi.org/10.1007/s11292-013-9189-9.

42. Leventhal T, Dupéré V. Moving to opportunity: does long-term exposure to "low-poverty" neighborhoods make a difference for adolescents? Soc Sci Med 2011;73(5):737–43. https://doi.org/10.1016/j.socscimed.2011.06.042.

43. Ejike CO, Woo H, Galiatsatos P, et al. Contribution of individual and neighborhood factors to racial disparities in respiratory outcomes. Am J Respir Crit Care Med 2021;203(8):987–97. https://doi.org/10.1164/rccm.202002-0253oc.

44. Sarcoidosis • AARDA. Available at: https://www.aarda.org/diseaseinfo/sarcoidosis/. Accessed April 26, 2021.

45. Hena KM. Sarcoidosis epidemiology: race matters. Front Immunol 2020;11(September):10–4.

46. Spagnolo P, Rossi G, Trisolini R, et al. Pulmonary sarcoidosis. Lancet Respir Med 2018;6(5): 389–402. https://doi.org/10.1016/S2213-2600(18)30064-X.

47. Harper LJ, Gerke AK, Wang XF, et al. Income and other contributors to poor outcomes in U.S. patients with sarcoidosis. Am J Respir Crit Care Med 2020; 201(8):955–64.

48. Rabin DL, Richardson MSA, Stein SR, et al. Sarcoidosis severity and socioeconomic status. Eur Respir J 2001;18(3):499–506. https://doi.org/10.1183/09031936.01.00056201.

49. Rabin DL, Thompson B, Brown KM, et al. Sarcoidosis: social predictors of severity at presentation. Eur Respir J 2004;24(4):601–8. https://doi.org/10.1183/09031936.04.00070503.

50. Gaffney AW, Woolhander S, Himmelstein D, et al. Disparities in pulmonary fibrosis care in the United States: an analysis from the Nationwide Inpatient Sample. BMC Health Serv Res 2018;18(1):1–8. https://doi.org/10.1186/s12913-018-3407-0.

51. Quon BS, Psoter K, Mayer-Hamblett N, et al. Disparities in access to lung transplantation for patients with cystic fibrosis by socioeconomic status. Am J Respir Crit Care Med 2012;186(10):1008–13. https://doi.org/10.1164/rccm.201205-0949OC.

52. Mathur AK, Schaubel DE, Gong Q, et al. Racial and ethnic disparities in access to liver transplantation. Liver Transpl 2010;16(9):1033–40. https://doi.org/10.1002/lt.22108.

53. Lederer DJ, Caplan-Shaw CE, O'Shea MK, et al. Racial and ethnic disparities in survival in lung transplant candidates with idiopathic pulmonary fibrosis. Am J Transpl 2006;6(2):398–403. https://doi.org/10.1111/j.1600-6143.2005.01205.x.

54. Kerem E, Cohen-Cymberknoh M. Disparities in cystic fibrosis care and outcome: Socioeconomic status and beyond. Chest 2016;149(2):298–300. https://doi.org/10.1016/j.chest.2015.08.021.

55. Oates GR, Baker E, Rowe SM, et al. Tobacco smoke exposure and socioeconomic factors are independent predictors of pulmonary decline in pediatric cystic fibrosis. J Cyst Fibros 2020;19(5):783–90. https://doi.org/10.1016/j.jcf.2020.02.004.

56. Harness-Brumley CL, Elliott AC, Rosenbluth DB, et al. Gender differences in outcomes of patients with cystic fibrosis. J Womens Heal 2014;23(12): 1012–20. https://doi.org/10.1089/jwh.2014.4985.

57. FitzSimmons SC. The changing epidemiology of cystic fibrosis. J Pediatr 1993;122(1):1–9. https://doi.org/10.1016/S0022-3476(05)83478-X.

58. Rosenfeld M, Davis R, FitzSimmons S, et al. Gender gap in cystic fibrosis mortality. Am J Epidemiol 1997; 145(9):794–803. https://doi.org/10.1093/oxfordjournals.aje.a009172.

59. Demko CA, Byard PJ, Davis PB. Gender differences in cystic fibrosis: Pseudomonas aeruginosa infection. J Clin Epidemiol 1995;48(8):1041–9. https://doi.org/10.1016/0895-4356(94)00230-N.

Disparities in Lung Transplantation

Simran K. Randhawa, MD[a],*, Sophia H. Roberts, MD[b], Varun Puri, MD, MSCI[c]

KEYWORDS

- Disparities • Lung transplantation • Donor • Recipient

KEY POINTS

- Lung transplantation has seen a steady growth and remains the standard of care for the treatment of end-stage lung disease.
- However, there exist various forms of disparities across all levels in lung transplantation.
- Disparities in the donor lung population are evident in the racial and gender distribution of donors.
- Similar disparities exist in the lung recipients and are compounded by differential geographic access.

According to the World Health Organization,[1] disparities are defined as "differences in health that are not only unnecessary and avoidable, but in addition, are considered unfair and unjust." Lung transplantation (LT) is a complex procedure with several potential barriers to access at sentinel time points, including accurate and prompt initial diagnosis, appropriate management of the pulmonary disease process, timely referral to a transplant center, pretransplant evaluation, registration to the waiting list, the transplant operation, and extensive post-transplant care. Through this article, we try to understand disparities in the area of LT and their impact on patient outcomes.

DISPARITIES IN LUNG DONORS
Importance of a Diverse Donor Population

Historically, in the United States, rates of deceased donor organ donation have been lower among racial and ethnic minority populations.[2] This leads to medical and logistical challenges because a more diverse donor registry is beneficial for many reasons. It gives ethnic minorities on the transplant waiting list a better chance to find a good donor match. In addition, the success of

organ transplantation and avoidance of organ rejection depends on the recipient's histocompatibility with the donated organ, Understandably, there is a greater degree of immunologic compatibility between donors and recipients from comparable ethnoracial communities. Furthermore, recipients with rare markers are more likely to match someone from a similar ethnic background.[3]

However, recent trends demonstrate that most organs for LT come from nonminority donors because of the disproportionate representation of ethnoracial minorities in the registered organ donor pool.[4] Cohort studies indicate that the authorization rate of African American families for deceased organ donation remains significantly lower than that of white families (54.9% vs 77.0%).[5] Callender and colleagues interviewed a cohort of 40 African Americans and identified 5 barriers to organ donation registration: lack of transplantation awareness, religious beliefs and misperceptions, distrust of the medical community, fear of premature declaration of death after signing a donor card, and fear of racism.[6] Additional factors acting as barriers to donor registration include cultural apprehension toward

[a] Division of Cardiothoracic Surgery, University of Colorado School of Medicine, Aurora, CO, USA; [b] Department of Surgery, Washington University School of Medicine, St Louis, MO, USA; [c] Division of Cardiothoracic Surgery, Washington University School of Medicine, St Louis, MO, USA
* Corresponding author: Washington University School of Medicine, Barnes-Jewish Hospital, Campus Box 8234 660 South Euclid Avenue, Saint Louis, MO 63110-1093.
E-mail address: randhawa.sk18@gmail.com

Thorac Surg Clin 32 (2022) 51–55
https://doi.org/10.1016/j.thorsurg.2021.09.001
1547-4127/22/© 2021 Elsevier Inc. All rights reserved.

discussing death in general, religious beliefs including that ones body must be whole to go to heaven, and distrust of the medical system.[7]

Over the past few decades, the transplant community has attempted to systematically engage minority communities and overcome these barriers to organ donation through a variety of interventions. Callender and colleagues have established The National Minority Organ Tissue Transplant Education Program (MOTTEP), a grassroots organization designed to (1) educate minority communities about organ transplantation; (2) empower minority communities to develop programs to increase awareness of organ donation; (3) increase minority engagement in organ transplantation by facilitating family discussions and organ donor registration; and (4) promote efforts for disease prevention to decrease the future need for transplantation.[6] Through culturally appropriate health education programs, the National MOTTEP has been able to significantly increase African American participants' reported trust in doctors, future plans to donate organs, and understanding of the need for organ donation.[8]

Knowledge of the allocation system and experiential knowledge of a transplant recipient have been shown to be critical aspects of the decision-making process for potential African American organ donors.[9] However, the manner in which potential donors and families of donors are approached is equally central to this decision. In a study comparing African American families who authorized or refused organ donation at the bedside, Siminoff and colleagues reported that African American families who authorized donation were more likely to cite excellent communication with the Organ Procurement Organization (OPO) requester as a factor that significantly influenced their decision. Such behaviors included the OPO requester listening carefully to the families, taking their concerns seriously, responding appropriately to these concerns, giving families adequate time to discuss and deliberate, responding to strong emotion with sensitivity and empathy.[10] This study highlights the importance of not only the content of information provided to individuals and families considering organ donation but also the culturally competent manner in which this information is relayed.

These endeavors have led to greater participation by minorities in organ donation over time. Between 1990 and 2008, African American organ donors per million (O.D.M) have increased from 8 O.D.M. to 53 O.D.M., and African Americans made up 15% of deceased organ donors in 2019.[6,11] In a recent study of the Scientific Registry for Transplant Recipients and the Centers for Disease Control and Prevention Wide-ranging Online Date for Epidemiologic Research Detailed Mortality File, Kernodle and colleagues observed a 1.6-fold increase in deceased organ donation among white individuals between 1999 and 2017.[12] Among Black and American Indian/Alaska Native individuals, the donation ratio increased 2.58-fold and 1.40-fold, respectively. However, overall black individuals are donating at 69% the rate of white individuals. These results suggest that although there are significant differences in donation rates across racial groups, these differences are diminishing over time. Continued efforts in outreach, education, and donor recruitment will be crucial to maintaining and expanding a diverse donor pool. One such avenue is to use social media as a sensor for organ donation awareness.[13] This has the potential to monitor organ donation awareness in real-time at a large-scale and to serve as a platform for delivering large-scale, community-based interventions to raise awareness while improving public attitudes and concern for a public health issue such as organ donation.

Sex-Based Disparities in Lung Donors

Despite 50.8% of the adult US population being composed of women,[14] there are significant sex-based differences in the organ donor pool. In a 2011 study, Murugan and colleagues found a 1.5-fold higher prevalence of registered male deceased organ donors over a 12-year period.[15] Similarly, the 2020 Organ Procurement and Transplantation Network (OPTN) report shows that 60% of donors were men.[11] Somewhat surprisingly, the proportion of male donors has been steadily increasing over the last 20 years.

Sex-associated differences in LT can potentially affect organ size match, metabolic demands of the organ, as well as circulating hormones, and a wide range of cellular receptors. The International Society for Heart and Lung Transplantation (ISHLT) Registry adult lung transplant report in 2004 noted that female to female LT was associated with a lower risk of 1-year mortality in a multivariate logistic regression model.[16] This suggests important sex-based biologic effects involving the interface between the donor organ and the recipient environment. Hence, it is imperative that necessary steps are taken to promote a more equal representation of women as lung donors. These interventions should be targeted toward changing attitudes, values, and beliefs pertaining to organ donation in the entire population, with a particular focus on female donors. These efforts can be accompanied by providing public access to sex-specific donor and recipient data and outcomes to highlight the advantages of concordant LT.

DISPARITIES IN LUNG TRANSPLANT RECIPIENTS

Disparities in LT extend to the recipient population as well. These barriers may be related to geography, race, or socioeconomic status.

Geographic Barriers to Access

In May 2005, the OPTN changed the policy for lung allocation for transplantation in the United States from a system that allocated donor lungs based primarily on waiting time to a system that allocated lungs based on a Lung Allocation Score (LAS).[17] The LAS is an adjusted scale from 0 to 100 based on disease severity and medical urgency, The LAS system is based on statistical models that aim to diminish predicted waitlist mortality and optimize post-transplantation 1-year survival. Though there is broad consensus that the LAS system has been a significant improvement over waiting list time-based allocation, the 2005 policy change, however, did not address the impact of geography on allocation. Transplant candidates were prioritized by LAS, but lungs were offered first to candidates within the boundaries of the donor's donation service area (DSA), thus bypassing candidates with a higher LAS outside the DSA. This led to a number of studies to explore geographic disparities in LT.[18,19] A national study by Kosztowski and colleagues used Scientific Registry of Transplant Recipients (SRTR) data to calculate lung transplant rates among more than 7000 waitlist candidates (ages 12 years or older).[20] They found that, even after adjusting for LAS and blood type, there was substantial evidence of DSA-level geographic disparity in LT. Candidates could more than double their rate of lung transplant by switching their DSA regions (median incidence rate ratio: 2.05).

In November 2017, in response to a lawsuit in the state of New York, focused on geographic inequity in lung allocation, an emergency change was made by UNOS to the lung allocation policy. This change eliminated the DSA as the first geographic tier of allocation and replaced it with a 250 nautical mile circle around the donor hospital. It was expected that this policy change would reduce geographic inequities in access to LT among waitlisted patients with the greatest severity of illness. However, initial reports have highlighted unanticipated logistical problems with a significant decline in local LT, greatly increased organ acquisition and travel costs, a higher organ discard rate, and a higher overall cost to the system.[21,22] Although the impact of the lung allocation policy in LT on geographic disparities remains largely conjectural, prior studies in LT have shown that broader sharing does not necessarily reduce geographic disparities.[23] Theoretic modeling suggests that perhaps combining DSAs into novel regions using mathematical redistricting optimization would reduce geographic disparities in transplantation rates.[24]

The OPTN allows transplant candidates within the United States to register for transplantation at more than one transplant center, a practice known as multiple listing. Multiple listing has been used as a strategy to overcome geographic inequities in access to transplantation, with migration of patients from areas of poor access to those with improved access. As expected, multiple listed candidates have a higher likelihood of receiving an LT than comparable single-listed candidates. Socioeconomic factors such as white race, higher education level, and private insurance have been associated with multiple listing in renal, liver, and heart transplant candidates.[25–28] Similarly, a national study using SRTR data showed that white candidates, candidates with a college or postcollege degree, and those with private insurance were more likely to be multiple listed for LT.[29] This suggests that multiple listing potentially allows socioeconomic status and physical mobility to prevail over medical acuity, thus standing at odds with the OPTN Final Rule's mandate. Although the complex debate over the merits, ethics, and propriety of multiple listing persist, it is prudent to evaluate and address geographic and other clinical disparities in LT access in order to decrease the need for multiple listing and improve the waitlist equity in lung transplant. Optimizing allocation policy to improve equity in access should remain a priority.

Sex-Based Disparities in Transplantation Rates

There is no convincing evidence indicating sex-based disparity in lung allocation in the United States. In the United Network for Organ Sharing (UNOS) transplant waitlist database, there are fewer women than men on the waiting list for kidney transplant (38% women), liver transplant (39% women), and heart transplant (only 24% women).[11] Conversely, women comprise 58% of candidates awaiting LT. In terms of graft survival, data suggest that women perform better than men, (5-year graft survival 55.6% vs 50.3% in men).[11] Reasons for these differences are likely multifactorial, including better compliance and overall knowledge and self-monitoring among women, but there is a lack of good-quality follow-up data.[30]

Racial Disparities in LT

Racial inequity refers to the social, financial, and structural disparities that affect different races within the United States. Such inequities may be manifested in the distribution of power, economic resources, and life opportunities afforded to people based on their race or ethnicity. Health care disparities in disease outcomes by racial, ethnic, and socioeconomic status have been widely reported in the literature. Those with higher incomes, better jobs, and more years of schooling tend to be healthier, have better outcomes after the onset of illness, and simply live longer.[31] Racial minority groups tend to have a significant comorbid disease burden, which may manifest as increased rates of end-organ failure and disproportionate representation on organ transplantation waiting lists.

Racial disparities in outcomes are well reported among patients with end-stage lung disease who are on the transplant waiting list. African American patients with end-stage lung disease have worse survival when compared with whites while on the lung transplant waiting list.[32,33] In their study of the UNOS database, Lederer and colleagues observed that after listing for LT, black patients with chronic obstructive pulmonary disease were less likely to undergo transplantation and more likely to die or be removed from the transplant list compared with white patients.[33] They found that differences in insurance coverage, socioeconomic status, and unequal access to care may have been some of the contributing factors to these differences. These findings indicate that transplant pulmonologists and surgeons should endeavor to list black patients with end-stage lung disease at the earliest appropriate time, as the likelihood of transplantation for black patients is lower than that of whites. However, such disparate outcomes fortunately do not extend to post-transplant survival rates. While in the historical era of LT, nonwhites had an increased risk of death compared with whites, this racial disparity has largely been eliminated in the modern era likely due, in part, to increasing awareness, and improved post-transplant quality of care.[34]

Socioeconomic Disparities in LT

In a study using data from the Cystic Fibrosis Foundation Patient Registry, Quon and colleagues examined the influence of socioeconomic status on access to LT in the United States.[35] They noted that Medicaid beneficiaries, those without a high school education, and those living in neighborhoods with a median household income below 200% of the federal poverty line (corresponding to about $34,000 per year for a family of four[36]) were less likely to be listed for LT even after accounting for differences in demographics, measures of disease severity, and potential contraindications. Additional studies have demonstrated a net transfer of lungs from low-income donors to high-income recipients in the United States.[37] Some issues affecting listing for LT among those with lower socioeconomic status include inadequate social support, fear of missing days at work for caregivers, and inadequate insurance coverage. Educating both providers and patients on these issues, avoiding referral delays, and patient-level support in the form of increasing home care services, enhancing transportation services, and lowering out-of-pocket drug costs may allay some of these specific problems.

SUMMARY

Significant ethnoracial and socioeconomic disparities impact the donor pool in LT as well access to LT in the United States. It has become increasingly important to address the issues of access and equity in LT. Close cooperation between the policymakers, the community, and medical professionals will be necessary to address disparities in LT to optimize access and outcomes.

DISCLOSURE

The authors have nothing to disclose.

REFERENCES

1. Whitehead M. The concepts and principles of equity and health. Int J Health Serv 1992;22(3):429–45.
2. Nathan HM, Conrad SL, Held PJ, et al. Organ donation in the United States. Am J Transplant 2003; 3(Suppl 4):29–40.
3. Kransdorf EP, Pando MJ, Gragert L, et al. HLA population genetics in solid organ transplantation. Transplantation 2017;101(9):1971–6.
4. Melanson TA, Hockenberry JM, Plantinga L, et al. New kidney allocation system associated with increased rates of transplants among black and hispanic patients. Health Aff (Millwood) 2017;36(6): 1078–85.
5. Goldberg DS, Halpern SD, Reese PP. Deceased organ donation consent rates among racial and ethnic minorities and older potential donors. Crit Care Med 2013;41(2):496–505.
6. Callender CO, Miles PV. Minority organ donation: the power of an educated community. J Am Coll Surg 2010;210(5):708–15, 715-7.
7. Irving MJ, Tong A, Jan S, et al. Factors that influence the decision to be an organ donor: a systematic

review of the qualitative literature. Nephrol Dial Transplant 2012;27(6):2526–33.

8. Callender CO, Hall MB, Branch D. An assessment of the effectiveness of the Mottep model for increasing donation rates and preventing the need for transplantation–adult findings: program years 1998 and 1999. Semin Nephrol 2001;21(4):419–28.

9. Jacob Arriola KR, Robinson DH, Perryman JP, et al. Understanding the relationship between knowledge and African Americans' donation decision-making. Patient Educ Couns 2008;70(2):242–50.

10. Siminoff LA, Alolod GP, Gardiner HM, et al. A comparison of the content and quality of organ donation discussions with african american families who authorize and refuse donation. J Racial Ethn Health Disparities 2021;8(2):485–93.

11. Available at: https://optn.transplant.hrsa.gov/data/view-data-reports/national-data/#. Accessed July 27, 2021.

12. Kernodle AB, Zhang W, Motter JD, et al. Examination of racial and ethnic differences in deceased organ donation ratio over time in the US. JAMA Surg 2021;156(4):e207083.

13. Murphy MD, Pinheiro D, Iyengar R, et al. A data-driven social network intervention for improving organ donation awareness among minorities: analysis and optimization of a cross-sectional study. J Med Internet Res 2020;22(1):e14605.

14. Available at: https://www.census.gov/quickfacts/fact/table/US/LFE046219. Accessed August 21, 2021.

15. Murugan R, Sileanu F, Wahed AS, et al. Sex differences in deceased donor organ transplantation rates in the United States. Transplantation 2011;92(11):1278–84.

16. Sato M, Gutierrez C, Kaneda H, et al. The effect of gender combinations on outcome in human lung transplantation: the International Society of Heart and Lung Transplantation Registry experience. J Heart Lung Transplant 2006;25(6):634–7.

17. Egan TM, Murray S, Bustami RT, et al. Development of the new lung allocation system in the United States. Am J Transplant 2006;6(5 Pt 2):1212–27.

18. Russo MJ, Meltzer D, Merlo A, et al. Local allocation of lung donors results in transplanting lungs in lower priority transplant recipients. Ann Thorac Surg 2013;95(4):1231–4. discussion: 1234-5].

19. Iribarne A, Meltzer DO, Chauhan D, et al. Distribution of donor lungs in the United States: a case for broader geographic sharing. Clin Transplant 2016;30(6):688–93.

20. Kosztowski M, Zhou S, Bush E, et al. Geographic disparities in lung transplant rates. Am J Transplant 2019;19(5):1491–7.

21. Available at: https://optn.transplant.hrsa.gov/media/2810/hr2018_01_analysis_report.pdf. Accessed April 23, 2021.

22. Puri V, Hachem RR, Frye CC, et al. Unintended consequences of changes to lung allocation policy. Am J Transplant 2019;19(8):2164–7.

23. Bowring MG, Zhou S, Chow EKH, et al. Geographic disparity in deceased donor liver transplant rates following share 35. Transplantation 2019;103(10):2113–20.

24. Gentry SE, Massie AB, Cheek SW, et al. Addressing geographic disparities in liver transplantation through redistricting. Am J Transplant 2013;13(8):2052–8.

25. Merion RM, Guidinger MK, Newmann JM, et al. Prevalence and outcomes of multiple-listing for cadaveric kidney and liver transplantation. Am J Transplant 2004;4(1):94–100.

26. Sanaei Ardekani M, Orlowski JM. Multiple listing in kidney transplantation. Am J Kidney Dis 2010;55(4):717–25.

27. Kohn R, Kratz JR, Markmann JF, et al. The migrated liver transplantation candidate: insight into geographic disparities in liver distribution. J Am Coll Surg 2014;218(6):1113–8.

28. Givens RC, Dardas T, Clerkin KJ, et al. Outcomes of multiple listing for adult heart transplantation in the United States: analysis of OPTN Data From 2000 to 2013. JACC Heart Fail 2015;3(12):933–41.

29. Mooney JJ, Yang L, Hedlin H, et al. Multiple listing in lung transplant candidates: a cohort study. Am J Transplant 2019;19(4):1098–108.

30. Norcross WA, Ramirez C, Palinkas LA. The influence of women on the health care-seeking behavior of men. J Fam Pract 1996;43(5):475–80.

31. Adler NE, Boyce T, Chesney MA, et al. Socioeconomic status and health. The challenge of the gradient. Am Psychol 1994;49(1):15–24.

32. Lederer DJ, Caplan-Shaw CE, O'Shea MK, et al. Racial and ethnic disparities in survival in lung transplant candidates with idiopathic pulmonary fibrosis. Am J Transplant 2006;6(2):398–403.

33. Lederer DJ, Benn EK, Barr RG, et al. Racial differences in waiting list outcomes in chronic obstructive pulmonary disease. Am J Respir Crit Care Med 2008;177(4):450–4.

34. Liu V, Weill D, Bhattacharya J. Racial disparities in survival after lung transplantation. Arch Surg 2011;146(3):286–93.

35. Quon BS, Psoter K, Mayer-Hamblett N, et al. Disparities in access to lung transplantation for patients with cystic fibrosis by socioeconomic status. Am J Respir Crit Care Med 2012;186(10):1008–13.

36. Department of Health and Human Services. Annual update of the HHS poverty guidelines. Available at: https://www.federalregister.gov/d/2021-01969. Accessed April 27, 2021.

37. Sehgal AR. The net transfer of transplant organs across race, sex, age, and income. Am J Med 2004;117(9):670–5.

Racial Disparities in Esophageal Cancer

Allan Pickens, MD

KEYWORDS

- Esophageal cancer • Squamous cell esophageal cancer • Esophageal adenocarcinoma • Race
- Racial disparity • Esophagectomy

KEY POINTS

- Advances in multimodal treatment have improved esophageal cancer outcomes.
- Surgical intervention for both esophageal squamous cell cancer and adenocarcinoma improves survival.
- Minorities have been reported to undergo fewer esophageal cancer resections and have the worst long-term survival.

INTRODUCTION

Esophageal cancer is one of the deadliest cancers worldwide. It is the ninth most common type of malignancy and the sixth leading cause of cancer deaths globally.[1] The 2 main histologic types of esophageal cancer, squamous cell carcinoma (ESCC) and adenocarcinoma (EAC), differ greatly in incidence and etiology. During the past four decades, important changes have occurred in the epidemiologic patterns associated with both types of esophageal cancer. Advances in the diagnosis, staging, and treatment of esophageal cancer have led to improvements in survival; however, the benefits have not been experienced equally across all races.

The incidence of EAC has increased in many Western societies, including North America, Europe, and Australia, whereas the incidence of ESCC has declined in these areas.[2] In the United States (US), there has been an alarming increase in the incidence of EAC and a decrease in ESCC. The rising incidence of esophageal cancer is the highest of any other malignancy in the United States. Worldwide, ESCC remains the predominant histologic type.[3]

Regarding gender and racial distribution, EAC is more common in men when compared with women (7:1 ratio), and its incidence rate is higher in Whites when compared with Blacks.[4] The incidence of EAC is 5-fold more common in Whites than in Blacks in the United States.[5] Risk factors for EAC may be divided into genetic and nongenetic components (**Table 1**). Clustering of EAC within several families has suggested the presence of a genetic component in EAC. The identification of this subset of patients has given rise to the term "familial EAC," which is also referred to as "familial Barrett esophagus." Familial EAC is defined as the presence of 2 or more family members diagnosed with Barrett esophagus, EAC, or gastroesophageal junction EAC.[6] Studies have shown that familial cases of EAC tend to develop at a younger age, and are less strongly associated with other risk factors for EAC.[7] Nongenetic risk factors are better established in the development of EAC and include Barrett esophagus, gastroesophageal reflux disease (GERD), obesity, and tobacco smoking. The prevalence of GERD in the Western population is about 10% to 20%; reflux is capable of producing EAC through preneoplastic Barrett esophagus. Barrett esophagus develops in 6% to 14% of patients with GERD and 0.5% to 1% will develop EAC.[7] For similar reasons, past use of lower esophageal sphincter-relaxing drugs is positively associated with the risk of EAC.

Despite the increasing incidence of EAC in the west, ESCC continues to be the most prevalent type of esophageal cancer worldwide as it accounts for 90% of all esophageal cancers each

thoracic.theclinics.com

Emory University, 550 Peachtree Street, NW, Davis Fisher Building, 4th Floor, Atlanta, GA 30308, USA
E-mail address: apicke3@emory.edu

Thorac Surg Clin 32 (2022) 57–65
https://doi.org/10.1016/j.thorsurg.2021.09.004

Table 1
Risk factors for squamous cell carcinoma and adenocarcinoma of the esophagus

Risk Factor	Squamous Cell Carcinoma	Adenocarcinoma
Geography	Southeastern Africa, Asia, Iran, South America	Western Europe, North America (United States), Australia
Race	Black > White	White > Black
Gender	Male > Female	Male > Female
Alcohol	++++	—
Tobacco	++++	++
Obesity	—	+++
GERD	—	++++
Diet: Low fruits and vegetables	++	+
Socioeconomic conditions	++	—
Genetic aspects	++	+

+, associated risk; —, no risk associated.

year.[8] Geographically, in contrast to EAC, ESCC is more commonly seen in developing countries. Specifically, the highest rates were observed in Eastern and South-East Asia, followed by sub-Saharan Africa and Central Asia. Similar to EAC, ESCC is more commonly seen in men.[9] Regarding ethnicity, ESCC has a higher incidence in Blacks when compared with other races (White, Pacific Islanders, American Indian, or Alaskan Natives).[9] Risk factors for ESCC include low socioeconomic status, tobacco smoking, and alcohol consumption (see **Table 1**). Both tobacco and alcohol appear to have a synergistic effect on increasing ESCC risk. Diet also plays a significant role in developing ESCC. Consumption of hot beverages, nitrosamine (seen in processed meats), red meat, and micronutrient deficiencies (beta-carotene, folate, vitamin C, vitamin E, and riboflavin) have all been linked with a higher risk of ESCC.[10] Achalasia, a motility disorder of the esophagus, confers an increased risk.[11] Similarly, caustic chemicals increase the risk of ESCC.[12] There are also conditions with a genetic basis, such as an autosomal dominant disease called tylosis, that are related to the development of ESCC. Plummer-Vinson syndrome is the triad of dysphagia, iron-deficiency anemia, and esophageal webs, and it correlates with a 10% increased likelihood of ESCC. Establishing an exact genetic component in the development of ESCC has been controversial. Risk factors are not the same for ESCC and EAC, but the risk of both histologic types increases with age, with a mean age of 67 years at diagnosis[13]

There is a paucity of data on the prevalence of esophageal cancer risk factors by race, ethnicity, and gender. ESCC has been confirmed to be more frequent among Blacks, and this higher prevalence has been attributed to an increased susceptibility to the carcinogenic effect of alcohol and tobacco.[5] According to the American Lung Association and the National Institute on Alcohol Abuse and Alcoholism, both tobacco and alcohol are more common in Whites[14,15]; yet, ESCC is more common in Blacks. This supports the concept of increased susceptibility to these agents by Blacks. Obesity is reported to increase EAC risk by increasing reflux.[16] Non-Hispanic Black adults (49.6%) had the highest prevalence of obesity compared with all other races according to the Centers for Disease Control and Prevention[17]; yet, Blacks are less likely to develop EAC. The risk factors do not clearly explain nor predict the racial disparity found in esophageal cancer.

Current literature suggests that the Black race is an independent risk factor for the development of ESCC.[8] In addition, Blacks have a higher likelihood of mortality when compared with other races.[18] A theory to explain this staggering disparity could be centered on socioeconomic status. Currently, ESCC has higher rates among populations in developing countries that have predominantly low socioeconomic status.[8] In addition, smoking, alcohol, and poor diet are known risk factors for the development of ESCC, and they are all risk factors that are less likely to be present in affluent, predominantly White populations. This is compounded by the innate distrust of doctors that exists within the Black community. Patients' health beliefs, risk aversion, treatment preferences, and cultural factors have been shown to influence health-seeking behaviors. Studies have shown that Black patients present with esophageal cancer at later stages than White patients.[19] This later

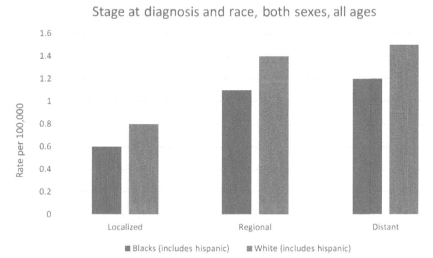

Fig. 1. Black patients are diagnosed with esophageal cancer at later stages; later stage presentation is associated with increased mortality. (*Data from* Cao J, Yuan P, Wang L, et al. Clinical Nomogram for Predicting Survival of Esophageal Cancer Patients after Esophagectomy. Sci Rep. 2016;6:26684.)

stage presentation by Blacks is concerning because studies have demonstrated that patients with a higher T stage have a poorer prognosis, independent of other factors.[20] (**Fig. 1**). The reasons for the late presentation are multifactorial, but later stage diagnosis results in fewer surgical options and an increased mortality rate for Blacks with esophageal cancer.

Screening

Early detection of esophageal cancer improves treatment options and outcomes, yet there are no standard or routine screening tests for esophageal cancer. In the United States, screening the general public for esophageal cancer is not recommended by any professional organization; recommendations only apply to high-risk persons (see **Table 1**). This is because no screening test has been shown to lower the risk of dying from esophageal cancer in average-risk people.

Barrett esophagus is the preneoplastic lesion preceding EAC; squamous dysplasia is the precursor lesion of ESCC. Both can be identified with effective screening.[21] Endoscopic screening of Barrett esophagitis for EAC is done. Endoscopic screening results in the detection of Barrett esophagitis in 6% to 12% of patients with prolonged GERD symptoms, most frequently White men over 50 years of age. A higher prevalence of reflux in Whites than other racial/ethnic groups in the United States has been reported.[22] The annual risk of EAC is approximately 1% for patients with low-grade dysplasia and 5% for patients with high-grade dysplasia. In 2016, the American

College of Gastroenterology recommended screening male patients with chronic GERD symptoms (>5 years), and 2 or more risk factors for Barrett esophagitis or EAC.[23] Multiple studies have supported the cost-effectiveness of endoscopic screening in this high-risk population.[24,25] The increasing prevalence of obesity and reflux parallels the increasing EAC incidence in White men.[26] Obesity correlates strongly with the changing epidemiology of EAC.

In contrast, endoscopic screening for ESCC is supposedly only cost-effective in areas of high incidence, such as in Northern and rural areas of China. The relatively high ESCC rates in Asians might be explained partly by exposures related to their traditional lifestyle. Such lifestyle risks include high consumption of processed meat and drinking high-temperature beverages.[27] In nonendemic areas such as the United States, screening has only been reported to be beneficial in certain diseases, not high-risk populations such as Black men. ESCC screening is recommended for patients with a history of head and neck cancers[28] and those with tylosis.[29] At this point, screening for ESCC is not recommended for Black men despite studies showing that ESCC disproportionately burdens Black men in the United States, and this cancer is frequently fatal in Black men. Effective screening for high-risk Black men has the potential to reduce mortality from this deadly disease. More research is needed to determine if screening is the key to reducing the racial disparity of ESCC for Black men.

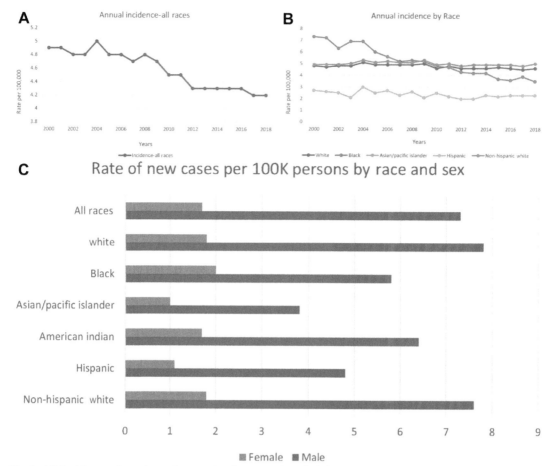

Fig. 2. (*A*) Incidence of esophageal cancer in all persons has slightly decreased. (*B*) The incidence of esophageal cancer according to race shows lower case numbers in Blacks compared with other races. (*C*) The rate of new esophageal cancer cases differs by race and sex. (*Data from* Esophagus Recent Trends in Relative Survival Rates, National Cancer Institute. Bethesda, MD, https://seer.cancer.gov, based on 2011- 2017 SEER data submission, Accessed April 2021.)

The American Cancer Society estimates 19,260 new esophageal cancer cases and 15,530 deaths from esophageal cancer in the United States in 2021.[30] The overall incidence of esophageal cancer among all Americans has slowly declined according to the Surveillance Epidemiology and End Results (SEER) database (**Fig. 2**A). Esophageal cancer has different trends in incidence rates across racial/ethnic groups (**Fig. 2**B). The decreasing incidence of ESCC in all groups parallels declining smoking prevalence. The more rapidly decreased smoking prevalence among Blacks is in line with the steep decline in the incidence of ESCC among Blacks.[31] EAC is predominately diagnosed in Whites.[32] The prevalence of abdominal obesity and increased reflux in Whites likely combine to produce the observed disparities in EAC incidence. The increasing prevalence of obesity and reflux parallels the increasing EAC

incidence in White men and women[33] (**Fig. 2**C). The observed racial and ethnic disparities in esophageal cancer rates and the temporal trends must be better defined to initiate effective interventions.

EVALUATION

Newly diagnosed esophageal cancer patients should undergo a complete history and physical examination, complete blood count, comprehensive chemistry profile, and upper GI endoscopy with biopsy of the primary tumor. Histologic evaluation is required for the correct diagnosis of ESCC or EAC. The extent of tumor involvement into the esophagogastric junction and cardia should be clearly documented. CT scan (with oral and intravenous contrast) of the chest and abdomen should also be performed. Endoscopic ultrasound and

FDG-PET/CT evaluation from skull base to mid-thigh are recommended if metastatic disease is not evident. Guidelines also recommend screening for a family history of esophageal cancer. Initial workup enables patients to be classified into 2 clinical-stage groups: locoregional cancer (stages I–III) and metastatic cancer (stage IV).[34]

TREATMENT

National Comprehensive Cancer Network (NCCN) and Society of Thoracic Surgeons (STS) guidelines for locoregional esophageal cancer (stages I–III) recommend surgical intervention in appropriately selected patients[35,36] as research has shown that surgical intervention offers the greatest survival benefit for early-stage disease as compared with chemoradiation alone.[37] Esophagectomy is indicated for medically fit patients with cT1b–cT2,N0 low-risk lesions. Endoscopic resection is appropriate for many T1a lesions. Primary treatment options for patients with cT1b–cT2,N+ or cT3-cT4a, any N tumors include preoperative chemoradiation, definitive chemoradiation (only for patients who decline surgery), perioperative chemotherapy, and preoperative chemotherapy. Definitive chemoradiation is the primary treatment option for patients with cT4b (unresectable) tumors.[38]

According to the SEER database review by Then and colleagues, most cases of esophageal cancer were treated with chemotherapy (61.7%), followed by radiotherapy (55.4%). Surgery was performed in only 26.6% of all patients with esophageal cancer. Patients with EAC were more likely to undergo surgical resection when compared with ESCC (32.9% vs 15.9%). Both EAC and ESCC patients underwent combined radiotherapy and chemotherapy at similar rates (45.8% vs 50.4%). Patients with EAC underwent combined surgical resection and chemotherapy at a higher rate than patients with ESCC (20.1% vs 9.3%). Similarly, triple therapy with surgery, radiotherapy, and chemotherapy was seen more frequently in patients with EAC than in patients with ESCC (17.8% vs 8.4%).[21]

Surgical intervention for both ESCC and EAC portends better outcomes. This finding has been validated by multiple studies. Using the SEER database, Abrams and colleagues showed that esophagectomy, when compared with chemoradiation, resulted in higher rates of 3-year survival for both ESCC and EAC.[39] Combining both chemoradiation and esophagectomy appears to be a more effective treatment modality. Sjoquist and colleagues conducted a meta-analysis containing data from 24 studies with a total of 4188 patients. They found that neoadjuvant chemoradiotherapy was superior to surgery alone in decreasing the risk of mortality.[40] Despite the strong evidence, the implementation of treatment regimens that include surgery appears to be impeded by cost-effectiveness. Salcedo and colleagues conducted a study evaluating cost. They found that chemoradiotherapy alone resulted in less cost for more quality-adjusted life years when compared with chemoradiotherapy combined with surgery.[41] The cost of including surgery in esophageal cancer treatment may be influencing the referral patterns and use of surgery for esophageal cancer, particularly in lower socioeconomic groups.

Lower rates of surgery have been identified in Black patients with esophageal cancer using the SEER database. Paulson and colleagues[42] found a significant underuse of esophagectomy for stages I, II, and III across all patient groups; however, in non-White and low socioeconomic patient cohorts, the underuse was even more pronounced. Steyerberg and colleagues[43] also reported that Black patients were half as likely to undergo esophageal cancer surgery, compared with White patients. Moreover, they found that not only were Black patients significantly less likely to be seen by a surgeon (70% vs 78%), but that even among patients seen by a surgeon, Black patients were significantly less likely to be offered surgical intervention (35% vs 59%).

Studies have consistently shown that minorities, including Blacks, are significantly less likely to receive care at high-volume hospitals for a variety of surgical procedures. Dubecz and colleagues[44] reported that overall, 44% of patients with esophageal cancer underwent esophagectomy; by comparison, more than 60% of the patients seen at specialized referral centers underwent surgical resection. Speicher and colleagues also reported that patients with esophageal cancer who travel longer distances to high-volume centers were more likely to undergo esophagectomy and had better outcomes than patients who stay close to home at low-volume centers.[45] Enhanced referral practices will ultimately increase the use of surgery to treat esophageal cancer.

Surgical resection is an essential part of curative treatment for esophageal cancer, but esophagectomy remains one of the most demanding surgical procedures, with significant associated morbidity and mortality.[46] Nevertheless, many patients seek definitive cancer care near home at their local community hospital rather than traveling to an unknown center of excellence in esophageal cancer care. Non-White patients may have decreased access to centers with sufficient volume and experience with complex esophageal operations.[47] The percentage of esophageal resections performed at high-volume hospitals significantly increased nationwide in the last decade, and the postoperative mortality rate dropped from 10.0% to 3.5% over 10 years. Small community hospitals have joined large academic centers so that the more complex procedures are performed in high-volume centers. Larger health care systems may not grant privileges for operations such as esophagectomies to surgeons who previously performed 1 or 2 per year. Finally, as the data on volume and outcome are publicly reported, individual surgeons may be more reluctant to perform operations linked to high morbidity and mortality for the fear of litigation. In response to the improved outcomes in larger-volume centers, the American Leapfrog group established a minimum hospital case volume of 13 esophageal resections for evidence-based hospital referral. The utilization of high-volume hospitals for esophagectomy has been associated with improved perioperative outcomes and reduced mortality.[48] Efforts should be made to understand factors influencing individual care decisions and improve referral practices to ensure optimal care is provided across all segments of the population, irrespective of race, insurance, or income status.

SURVEILLANCE

After esophageal cancer treatment, all patients should be followed systematically. However, surveillance strategies after successful local therapy for esophageal cancers remain controversial, with no high-level evidence to guide the development of algorithms that balance benefits and risks. In general, follow-up for asymptomatic patients should include a complete history and physical examination every 3 to 6 months for the first 2 years, every 6 to 12 months for years 3 to 5, and then annually thereafter. Laboratories, endoscopy with

biopsy, and imaging studies should be performed as clinically indicated.[34]

Participation in surveillance can be influenced by socioeconomic status. Insured patients tend to be more compliant with recommended follow-up. Blacks, Hispanics, and some Asian populations, when compared with Whites, appear to have lower levels of health insurance coverage according to the Institute of Medicine.[49] Universal health care would likely improve this statistic.

SURVIVAL

Overall, the 5-year survival rate of esophageal cancer, of all types, remains poor at approximately 20%. Esophageal cancer is found at the localized stage (T1-3, N0, M0), in only 25% of patients.[50] This stage of esophageal cancer is typically evaluated for surgery. Despite its poor prognosis, significant strides in esophageal cancer treatment have resulted in a decreased mortality over the past four decades. Age-adjusted death rates for esophageal cancer have been falling on average 1.2% each year over 2009 to 2018. When analyzing survival rates of esophageal cancer by type, EAC has a better prognosis when compared with ESCC. One study found that the 5-year relative survival rate of EAC increased from 5.7 to 13.6 during the study period. Similarly, the 5-year relative survival rate of ESCC increased from 4.5 to 11.8.[51]

Advances in multimodal treatment have improved esophageal cancer outcomes. However, not all populations have benefited from these treatment strategies, and survival continues to be poorer among minority patients[19] (**Fig. 3**). Nationally, Black patients with esophageal cancer have a 5-year survival rate of 13.7% compared with White patients with esophageal cancer, who have a 5-year survival rate of 20.6%.[52] Although differences in biology may play a role in these

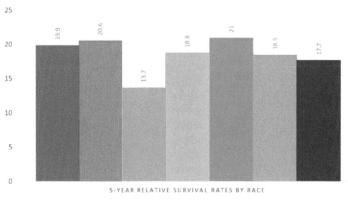

Fig. 3. The 5-year survival for Blacks is worst compared with other races. (*Data from* Esophagus Recent Trends in Relative Survival Rates, National Cancer Institute. Bethesda, MD, https://seer.cancer. gov, based on 2011- 2017 SEER data submission, Accessed April 2021.)

5-YEAR RELATIVE SURVIVAL RATES BY RACE

■ All races ■ White ■ Black ■ Hispanic ■ Non-hispanic ■ American indian ■ Asian/pacific islander

racial survival disparities, variation in the receipt of certain treatment options and access to health care are major contributors. Prior studies involving patients with esophageal and other cancer types have shown that race/ethnicity are predictors of whether patients receive cancer-directed surgery.[42] Potential explanations for the lower likelihood that racial minorities receive cancer-directed surgery have included theories suggesting that these patients' lower socioeconomic status, higher comorbidities, and decreased access to care are involved.[53]

According to Revels and colleagues, rates of resection for patients with midesophageal cancers (both ESCC and EAC) were low for all race/ethnicity groups; however, differences were particularly pronounced among Black patients with EAC. Only 15% of Black patients with midesophageal cancers underwent esophagectomy compared to 23% of Hispanics and 28.9% of Whites.[54] It is plausible that disparities in resection rates are more pronounced in Black patients because of the higher proportion of ESCC and therefore midesophageal tumors among this group. The undisputed increased incidence of ESCC in Black patients does not fully explain the paucity of surgical intervention. Black patients with EAC were also less likely to have surgery. As surgery correlates with improved esophageal cancer survival, the underuse of cancer-directed surgery in non-White patients contributes to higher mortality rates among this population. Accounting for patient-level factors and access-related issues have failed to fully explain the underuse of surgical resection and the excess mortality observed in non-White patients with esophageal cancer. Examination of physician attitudes, behaviors, and referral patterns may provide insight into changing practice patterns and assuring that non-White patients are referred to experienced surgeons for appropriate management of their esophageal cancer.

Disparities in resection rates and survival may also be related to the quality of care received and the race-related differences in the patient-physician relationship.[55] These issues must be clarified to better understand underlying causes for low esophagectomy rates in non-White patients with potentially resectable disease. Many minority individuals have cancer beliefs and attitudes that differ from those of nonminorities,[56] and these factors may be associated with the observed disparities in diagnosis and treatment. Mismatch of cultural beliefs, values, and experiences may limit the quality of the communication between some minority patients and their nonminority providers, thereby contributing to disparities

in the quality of health.[57] Finally, aspects of the health care system, such as available services and financial requirements, may exert different effects on esophageal cancer diagnosis and treatment, particularly for racial and ethnic minorities.[58] To decrease disparities in esophageal cancer outcomes, it will be necessary to understand the underlying causes for low esophagectomy rates in non-White patients and develop interventions that improve curative surgery rates. Diagnosis at an earlier stage and higher rates of surgery among minority patients with esophageal cancer could reduce the survival disparity.

Investigation into the role of race in treatment decisions and hospital-level factors that affect disease management is urgently needed. Studies using various large population-based data sets, including SEER, NCDB, Nationwide Inpatient Sample, National Surgical Quality Improvement Program, and The Society of Thoracic Surgeons databases have decisively shown that the Black race is a significant predictor of major morbidity, mortality, and overall survival.[59] Simply removing barriers to access will not fix the problem; in addition, we must find ways to engage vulnerable patients to facilitate their inclusion in the most effective care plans. Strategies to improve communication and gain the trust of these patients with cancer must be identified and implemented. In the meantime, improved education of patients and providers regarding treatment guidelines to ensure receipt of surgery in appropriate surgical candidates may improve outcomes for minority patients with esophageal cancer.

CLINICS CARE POINTS

- Early detection of esophageal cancer improves treatment options and outcomes.
- Barrett esophagus is the preneoplastic lesion preceding esophageal adenocarcinoma; squamous dysplasia is the precursor lesion of esophageal squamous cell cancer.
- Esophageal squamous cell cancer is more commonly diagnosed in Blacks; esophageal adenocarcinoma is more commonly found in Whites.
- Advances in multimodal treatment have improved esophageal cancer outcomes.
- Surgical intervention for both esophageal squamous cell cancer and adenocarcinoma portends better outcomes.

- Black patients have been reported to undergo fewer esophageal cancer resections and have the worst long-term survival.

DISCLOSURE

The author has nothing to disclose.

REFERENCES

1. Global Burden of Disease Cancer Collaboration, Fitzmaurice C, Dicker D, et al. The global burden of cancer 2013. JAMA Oncol 2015;1(4):505–27.
2. Rustgi AK, El-Serag HB. Esophageal carcinoma. N Engl J Med 2014;371(26):2499–509.
3. Pera M, Manterola C, Vidal O, et al. Epidemiology of esophageal adenocarcinoma. J Surg Oncol 2005;92(3):151–9.
4. Lagergren J. Adenocarcinoma of oesophagus: what exactly is the size of the problem and who is at risk? Gut 2005;54(Suppl 1):i1–5.
5. Baquet CR, Commiskey P, Mack K, et al. Esophageal cancer epidemiology in blacks and whites: racial and gender disparities in incidence, mortality, survival rates and histology. J Natl Med Assoc 2005;97:1471–8.
6. Van Nistelrooij AM, Dinjens WN, Wagner A, et al. Hereditary factors in esophageal adenocarcinoma. Gastrointest Tumors 2014;1(2):93–8.
7. Coleman HG, Xie SH, Lagergren J. The epidemiology of esophageal adenocarcinoma. Gastroenterology 2018;154(2):390–405.
8. Abnet CC, Arnold M, Wei WQ. Epidemiology of esophageal squamous cell carcinoma. Gastroenterology 2018;154(2):360–73.
9. Arnold M, Soerjomataram I, Ferlay J, et al. Global incidence of esophageal cancer by histological subtype in 2012. Gut 2015;64(3):381–7.
10. Liang H, Fan JH, Qiao YL. Epidemiology, etiology, and prevention of esophageal squamous cell carcinoma in China. Cancer Biol Med 2017;14(1):33–41.
11. Torres-Aguilera M, Remes Troche JM. Achalasia and esophageal cancer: risks and links. Clin Exp Gastroenterol 2018;11:309–16.
12. Zhang X, Wang M, Han H, et al. Corrosive induced carcinoma of esophagus after 58 years. Ann Thorac Surg 2012;94:2103–5.
13. Daly JM, Fry WA, Little AG, et al. Esophageal cancer: results of an American College of Surgeons Patient Care Evaluation Study. J Am Coll Surg 2000;190:562–72.
14. American Lung Association. Tobacco use in racial and ethnic populations. Available at: https://www.lung.org/. Accessed April 9, 2021.
15. NIH on alcohol abuse and alcoholism. Available at: http://www.niaaa.nih.gov/. Accessed April 9, 2021.
16. Kubo A, Corley DA. Body mass index and adenocarcinomas of the esophagus or gastric cardia: a systematic review and meta-analysis. Cancer Epidemiol Biomarkers Prev 2006;15:872–8.
17. CDC. Obesity. Available at: https://www.cdc.gov/. Accessed April, 2021.
18. Chen Z, Ren Y, Du XL, et al. Incidence and survival differences in esophageal cancer among ethnic groups in the United States. Oncotarget 2017;8(29):47037–51.
19. Greenstein AJ, Litle VR, Swanson SJ, et al. Racial disparities in esophageal cancer treatment and outcomes. Ann Surg Oncol 2008;15:881–8.
20. Cao J, Yuan P, Wang L, et al. Clinical nomogram for predicting survival of esophageal cancer patients after esophagectomy. Sci Rep 2016;6:26684.
21. Then EO, Lopez M, Saleem S, et al. Esophageal cancer: an updated surveillance epidemiology and end results database analysis. World J Oncol 2020;11(2):55–64.
22. El-Serag HB, Petersen NJ, Carter J, et al. Gastroesophageal reflux among different racial groups in the United States. Gastroenterology 2004;126(7):1692–9.
23. Shaheen NJ, Falk GW, Iyer PG, et al. ACG clinical guideline: diagnosis and management of Barrett's esophagus. Am J Gastroenterol 2016;111(1):30–50.
24. Gerson LB, Groeneveld PW, Triadafilopoulos G. Cost-effectiveness model of endoscopic screening and surveillance in patients with gastroesophageal reflux disease. Clin Gastroenterol Hepatol 2004;2(10):868–79.
25. Inadomi JM, Sampliner R, Lagergren J, et al. Screening and surveillance for Barrett esophagus in high-risk groups: a cost-utility analysis. Ann Intern Med 2003;138(3):176–86.
26. Wang Y, Beydoun MA. The obesity epidemic in the United States—gender, age, socioeconomic, racial/ethnic, and geographic characteristics: a systematic review and meta- regression analysis. Epidemiol Rev 2007;29:6–28.
27. Islami F, Boffetta P, Ren JS, et al. High-temperature beverages and foods and esophageal cancer risk—a systematic review. Int J Cancer 2009;125(3):491–524.
28. Su YY, Chen WC, Chuang HC, et al. Effect of routine esophageal screening in patients with head and neck cancer. JAMA Otolaryngol Head Neck Surg 2013;139(4):350–4.
29. Risk JM, Mills HS, Garde J, et al. The tylosis esophageal cancer (TOC) locus: more than just a familial cancer gene. Dis Esophagus 1999;12(3):173–6.
30. American Cancer Society. Key statistics for esophageal cancer. Available at: https://www.cancer.org/. Accessed April 23, 2021.
31. Jamal A, Homa DM, O'Connor E, et al. Current cigarette smoking among adults—United States, 2005–

2014. MMWR Morb Mortal Wkly Rep 2015;64(44): 1233–40.

32. Thrift AP, Whiteman DC. The incidence of esophageal adenocarcinoma continues to rise: analysis of period and birth cohort effects on recent trends. Ann Oncol 2012;23:3155–62.

33. Petrick JL, Nguyen T, Cook MB. Temporal trends of esophageal disorders by age in the Cerner Health Facts database. Ann Epidemiol 2016;26(2):151–4. e4.

34. Journal of the national comprehensive cancer network. Available at: https://jnccn.org/. Accessed April 23, 2021.

35. Little AG, Lerut AE, Harpole DH, et al. The Society of Thoracic Surgeons practice guidelines on the role of multimodality treatment for cancer of the esophagus and gastroesophageal junction. Ann Thorac Surg 2014;98(5):1880–5.

36. Ajani JA, Barthel JS, Bentrem DJ, et al. Esophageal and esophagogastric junction cancers. J Natl Compr Canc Netw 2011;9(8):830–87.

37. Steffen T, Dietrich D, Schnider A, et al. Recurrence patterns and long-term results after induction chemotherapy, chemoradiotherapy, and curative surgery in patients with locally advanced esophageal cancer. Ann Surg 2019;269(1):83–7.

38. Ajani JA, D'Amico TA, Bentrem DJ, et al. Esophageal and Esophagogastric Junction Cancers, Version 2.2019. J Natl Compr Canc Netw 2019;17(7): 855–83.

39. Abrams JA, Buono DL, Strauss J, et al. Esophagectomy compared with chemoradiation for early-stage esophageal cancer in the elderly. Cancer 2009; 115(21):4924–33.

40. Sjoquist KM, Burmeister BH, Smithers BM, et al. Survival after neoadjuvant chemotherapy or chemoradiotherapy for resectable esophageal carcinoma: an updated meta-analysis. Lancet Oncol 2011; 12(7):681–92.

41. Salcedo J, Suen SC, Bian SX. Cost-effectiveness of chemoradiation followed by esophagectomy versus chemoradiation alone in squamous cell carcinoma of the esophagus. Cancer Med 2020;9(2):440–6.

42. Paulson EC, Ra J, Armstrong K, et al. Underuse of esophagectomy as treatment for resectable esophageal cancer. Arch Surg 2008;143:1198–203.

43. Steyerberg EW, Earle CC, Neville BA, et al. Racial differences in surgical evaluation, treatment, and outcome of locoregional esophageal cancer: a population-based analysis of elderly patients. J Clin Oncol 2005;23:510–7.

44. Dubecz A, Sepesi B, Salvador R, et al. Surgical resection for locoregional esophageal cancer is underutilized in the United States. J Am Coll Surg 2010;211:754–61.

45. Speicher PJ, Englum BR, Ganapathi AM, et al. Traveling to a high-volume center is associated with

46. Sauvanet A, Mariette C, Thomas P, et al. Mortality and morbidity after resection for adenocarcinoma of the gastroesophageal junction: predictive factors. J Am Coll Surg 2005;201:253–62.

47. Bach PB, Pham HH, Schrag D, et al. Primary care physicians who treat blacks and whites. N Engl J Med 2004;351:575–84.

48. Birkmeyer JD, Stukel TA, Siewers AE, et al. Surgeon volume and operative mortality in the United States. N Engl J Med 2003;349(22):2117–27.

49. Bulatao RA, Anderson NB, editors. Understanding racial and ethnic differences in health in late life: a research Agenda. National research Council (US) panel on race, ethnicity, and health in later life. Washington (DC): National Academies Press (US); 2004.

50. Esophagus recent trends in relative survival rates, National Cancer Institute. Bethesda, MD. Available at: https://seer.cancer.gov. based on 2011- 2017 SEER data submission, Accessed April 23, 2021.

51. Polednak AP. Trends in survival for both histologic types of esophageal cancer in US surveillance, epidemiology and end results areas. Int J Cancer 2003;105(1):98–100.

52. National Cancer Institute. Surveillance, Epidemiology, and End Results Program (SEER), cancer statistics: esophageal cancer. Available at: https://seer.cancer.gov/statfacts/html/esoph.html. based on 2011-2017 SEER data submission, Accessed April 23, 2021.

53. Birkmeyer NJ, Gu N, Baser O, et al. Socioeconomic status and surgical mortality in the elderly. Med Care 2008;46:893–9.

54. Revels SL, Morris AM, Reddy RM, et al. Racial disparities in esophageal cancer outcomes. Ann Surg Oncol 2013;20:1136–41.

55. Manfredi C, Kaiser K, Matthews AK, et al. Are racial differences in patient–physician cancer communication and information explained by background, predisposing, and enabling factors? J Health Commun 2010;15:272–92.

56. Margolis ML, Christie JD, Silvestri GA, et al. Racial differences pertaining to a belief about lung cancer surgery: results of a multicenter survey. Ann Intern Med 2003;139:558–63.

57. Van Ryn M, Burke J. The effect of patient race and socio-economic status on physicians' perceptions of patients. Soc Sci Med 2000;50:813–28.

58. Davis TC, Williams MV, Marin E, et al. Health literacy and cancer communication. CA Cancer J Clin 2002; 52:134–49.

59. Rehmani SS, Liu B, Al-Ayoubi AM, et al. Racial disparity in utilization of high-volume hospitals for surgical treatment of esophageal cancer. Ann Thorac Surg 2018;106:346–53.

Challenges in the Methodology for Health Disparities Research in Thoracic Surgery

Sakib M. Adnan, MD[a], Michael Poulson, MD[b], Virginia R. Litle, MD[c], Cherie P. Erkmen, MD[d],*

KEYWORDS

• Health disparities • Population studies • Methodology • Equity • Marginalized groups

KEY POINTS

- There is considerable bias in health disparities research, largely as a result of heterogenous study design.
- Establishing the core definitions of health disparities, equity, and marginalized groups may help to limit bias in population-based studies.
- Awareness of the heterogeneity of data sources and data collection methods is needed to reduce barriers to accurate downstream data analysis and interpretation.
- Consideration of these factors is needed for high-quality study design, as health disparities research in thoracic surgery is still under development.

INTRODUCTION

A major goal in US public health is to eliminate disparities in health and health care, as addressed in the Health and Human Services' *Healthy People 2010* initiative.[1] Several health care organizations have since highlighted disparities as a focus of their research missions, with many potential summary measures proposed to bridge the gap in health disparities.[2,3] Most conclusions in health disparities research arise from large population-based studies, which bring potential selection biases when defining disparities and in the overall framework of population study designs. Similarly, faulty conclusions from biased interpretations of data can perpetuate disparities by failing to highlight the true discriminatory cause. Health differences are evident in the surgical literature, with several groups advocating for conscious study design with awareness of implicit and selection biases.[4–6] However, there is a paucity in literature in methodological strategy to limit these biases in population studies for health disparities, especially in the surgical community. The authors' aim is to describe the methodological issues in health disparities research within thoracic surgery and to offer proposals to reduce the bias associated with current approaches to disparities investigations.

ESTABLISHING DEFINITIONS AND CLARITY FOR APPLICATION: HEALTH DISPARITIES, EQUITY, AND MARGINALIZED POPULATIONS
Health Disparities

The basis of current health disparities research is the comparative study of differences in health outcomes between a proposed marginalized group

[a] Department of Surgery, Einstein Healthcare Network, 5401 Old York Road, Suite 510, Philadelphia, PA 19141, USA; [b] Department of Surgery, Boston Medical Center, Boston University School of Medicine, Boston, MA, USA; [c] Intermountain Healthcare, 5169 So. Cottonwood Street, Suite 640, Murray, UT 84107, USA; [d] Thoracic Medicine and Surgery, Temple University Hospital, 3401 N. Broad Street, Suite 501, Philadelphia, PA 19140, USA
* Corresponding author.
E-mail address: cherie.erkmen@tuhs.temple.edu

Thorac Surg Clin 32 (2022) 67–74
https://doi.org/10.1016/j.thorsurg.2021.09.008
1547-4127/22/© 2021 Elsevier Inc. All rights reserved.

and a less marginalized group. Although this design is largely accepted and appears conceptually simple, there is variance in defining a health disparity, and the selection of comparison groups is often based on assumption. These areas of inconsistency not only obscure the complexities of the many social determinants of health (SDH) but also reveal a need for a deeper understanding for methodological differences in defining and measuring health disparities.[7]

To offer clarity, the latest Health and Human Services initiative, *Healthy People 2020*, proposed a definition for a health disparity as "a particular type of health difference that is closely linked with economic, social, or economic disadvantage."[8] This definition offers a distinction between a health disparity and health difference, where the former hinges on a fundamental disadvantage, not just a difference based on grouping. Disparities have historically been linked to race, socioeconomic status (SES), and disability; however, ambiguity in the specific definition of a health disparity detracts from accurate and appropriately directed conclusions and resources.[9]

A more quantitative definition of a health disparity has been proposed by Keppel and colleagues[10] as the quantitative difference (rate, percentage, mean, and so forth) that separates a group from a specific reference point on a measure of health. Although this rather objective definition offers a framework for direct measurement of disparities, disparities are more heterogeneous in population-based comparative studies in the surgical literature. This was addressed as a primary concern in the 2015 National Institutes of Health and American College of Surgeons Summit, where the prevalence of nonstandard definitions of health disparities was thought to preclude complete linking of disparate data sets for accurate analysis.[11] Moreover, the clinicians in this summit proposed further research into implementing working quality metrics and more objective terms in future health disparities research. The adoption of more objective, measurable definitions in health disparities research is ongoing, with the anticipation that it may offer conclusions with greater external validity.

Health Equity

It is important to explicitly differentiate health disparities from health equity. Ambiguity in definitions may confound data, interpretation, and future interventions, including resource allocation to nondisadvantaged groups. Health disparities lie in a status of unequal health potential, and health equity is the goal of opportunity for everyone to attain

their highest level of health.[9] Health equity has been defined as a commitment toward fair distribution of health outcomes, resources, and its determinants across all groups in a population, regardless of social standing.[10] An extension of this definition was introduced in the *Healthy People 2010* initiative, which asserted that health equity can only be achieved through special efforts to improve the health of socially or economically disadvantaged groups.[11] Implicit in this definition is a component of social justice in defining health equity. The *Healthy People 2020* initiative further proposed that clarity in health equity might be provided by more bivariate approaches in research methodology. Specifically, this involves a measurement of health jointly in relation to a grouped attribute (income, education, race, and so forth), as opposed to a more univariate approach in which health is measured across individuals in a population regardless of associated attributes.[12] The major transition from this initiative to the *Healthy People 2030* initiative was a focus on more diverse metrics and measurement strategies to better elucidate upstream socioeconomic determinant of health.[13] Although a large body of recent health disparities research in surgery continues to rely on multivariate analyses, the exact methodological challenges to limit value judgements remain.[14,15] Still, awareness of these challenges in study design and its implications remain important, as they may guide health strategies and policies that have the potential to influence population health toward equity.

Marginalized Groups

Inherent in defining and evaluating health disparities is consideration of which populations would be considered marginalized. Marginalized populations are commonly defined based on race, ethnicity, or SES alone, with an extensive body of thoracic surgical literature describing the health inequity experienced by minorities and those with lower SES. For instance, a retrospective review of 7498 patients from the National Cancer Data Base (NCDB) demonstrated that black patients with thymic malignancies were more likely to have a lower median income, were less likely to receive surgical therapy, and were more likely to experience delays in surgical care than white patients.[16] Another retrospective cohort study reported that socioeconomically disadvantaged patients with early-stage non–small cell lung cancer were less likely to receive standard-of-care therapy and experienced poorer survival.[17] However, it is important to note that marginalization is based in preclusion from social mobility, leading to lower SES.[18]

The health inequities experienced by these established marginalized groups are reported across the surgical literature; however, many of these studies rely on binary or inconsistent definitions of "marginalized populations." Several groups advocate for clarification and standardization of this definition, especially in regards to race and SES.[19,20] Broader definitions have emerged in recent literature, with the interplay of SES, social class, and history of discrimination suggested as more accurate descriptors of marginalized groups.[21,22] However, challenges remain in developing objective measures of these factors. For instance, education, income, and employment serve as more superficial proxies for social class, which may change over the course of time and are differentially tied to racial and other marginalized groups based on historical preclusion from social mobility.[18] Furthermore, the intersection of disparities adds a level of complexity to data interpretation. Intersectionality is a framework based in critical race theory that emphasizes compounding marginalization with intersecting identities based in social constructs.[23] For example, differences in gender, gender identity, race, immigration status, disability, sexual orientation, and social status cannot simply be added or multiplied because these factors may be dependent on each other, nor can they be thought of as monoliths in and of themselves. Investigating health disparities requires an intersectional approach that integrates complex relationships between marginalized groups as well as the context of how power structures and vulnerability may change over time.[24] The challenge in defining marginalized groups remains because of its multifactorial nature, which should be a consideration in devising health disparities studies.

MEASUREMENT OF DISPARITIES AND SUBSEQUENT ANALYSES: SOURCES OF BIAS IN STUDY DESIGN
Data Sources

Health disparities and outcomes research has been performed for many decades, although more recently large clinical registries and administrative databases have become used for thoracic surgical research. With the continued evolution of health disparities research, it is crucial for researchers and the community to understand the strengths and limitations of these sources of data, and how they may affect the derived conclusions from a practical and ethical standpoint.

The NCDB is one of the most commonly used data sources for health disparities and outcomes research. This hospital-based registry captures approximately 70% of newly diagnosed cancer cases in the United States each year and allows for robust outcomes analyses.[25] However, the NCDB includes data from patients treated only at Commission of Cancer–accredited hospitals. This introduces an inherent selection bias, as patients with lower SES and in minority groups are less likely to be treated at these institutions. The demographic data within the NCDB, while extensive, are also less detailed within each variable and have stringent cutoff values making granular analyses limited.[26] Given that it is not a population-based registry, broader conclusions regarding health disparities cannot be fully asserted through use of the NCDB.

The National Surgical Quality Improvement Program (NSQIP) database includes voluntarily reported data across more than 600 sites in the United States. This cross-sectional data set includes broad demographic and outcomes data on general, vascular, and cardiothoracic surgeries. Similar to the NCDB, a major strength of the NSQIP is the breadth of available patient data, specifically for preexisting preoperative patient conditions and postoperative complications. However, data abstraction is limited to roughly 25% of all procedures performed at participating sites. The NSQIP also uses surgical clinical reviewers who retrospectively collect data, oftentimes with limited detail on demographic and case information. In addition, given that the focus of the NSQIP is on perioperative complications, only 30-day outcomes are reported, making generalized and long-term conclusions limited.[27]

The Society of Thoracic Surgeons (STS) database initially only recorded cardiac surgical outcomes, but expanded to general thoracic procedures in 2002, collecting data on 100% of all operations performed at more than 150 participating centers. Since then, the goal of the STS General Thoracic Surgery Database (STS-GTSD) has been 2-fold: quality improvement and health services research. It provides extensive and comprehensive demographic and preoperative data permitting analyses of more complete and accurate information. It has been reported as the largest and most comprehensive database for general thoracic surgery, although the limitations in disparities analysis using the STS database are inherent to its previous data collection methodology.[28] A revised data collection strategy has been proposed to reduce the burden of data entry and degree of input variable redundancy and discrepancy. With multiple limitations, the STS-

GTSD currently remains the largest thoracic surgery database in the United States for health services and disparities research.[29]

The Surveillance, Epidemiology, and End Results (SEER) database is a population-based cancer data set of 21 US registries that encompass a diverse sample of the population. The SEER database is a prominent source of health services information, given its large size and extensive epidemiologic data, with more than 40,000 publications referenced since its inception.[30] However, there is no report on patient education level, income, comorbidities, or functional status, factors that are requisite for providing detailed assertions on thoracic surgery health disparities.

Given the heterogeneity and weaknesses in each of the aforementioned databases, caution should be practiced during study design and methodology for general thoracic surgery disparities research. Attention should be directed toward the data source of interest, ensuring that the research question can be accurately answered with the available data. This requires understanding of the nuances and heterogeneity between the many available data sources.

Data Collection

Population-based disparities research relies on data collection from prospectively maintained data sets extrapolated from census reports or from patient-reported outcomes. These data can be challenging to collect, largely because of the diversity of input variables (ie, income, ZIP code, education level) used in the geocoding framework for disparities research. These variables serve as proxies for SES and often represent disparities across geographically distinct populations, as opposed to individual patients, and may lead to inaccurate conclusions.

However, this form of data collection, which is widely used, does offer strong evidence that those with lower SES or in more rural areas receive quality care and screening measures less often than those in higher SES groups. Specifically, several reports have suggested that minority and disadvantaged groups are less likely to receive lung cancer screening and first-line therapy.[31–35] However, few if any have explicitly linked SES to race, sex, or other marginalized identity. There is also evidence that these groups have less participation and engagement in research, largely because of patient-related factors, such as disease awareness, cost concerns, insurance coverage, and poor access to screening/treatment.[36] For health disparities research to expand in thoracic surgery, understanding of the complexities of data collection strategies, largely patient barriers, should be considered.

Data Analysis

A larger methodological issue exists in the large database studies, from which many conclusions of surgical disparities are drawn from. Demographic variables are often offered in binary terms, simplifying subsequent analysis at the expense of accuracy and generalizability. Similarly, there is a lack of breadth of patient information to address disparities based on marginalization owing to lesbian, gay, bisexual, transgender, and queer (LGBTQ+), disability, and immigration status, among others. Unique input variables in many data sets, which largely are used for secondary analyses, are often mistakenly used as variables for disparities research. This may involve proxy variables or microdata linkage for missing variables, or even the use of inferred variables to impute information for missing information.[37,38] Furthermore, the population of minority patients is oftentimes, by nature, much smaller than that of nonminority patients, increasing the chance of error in many reported outcomes in these studies.[39] Although some of these methodological concerns may be difficult to control, caution should be exercised when structuring the design for population-based studies.

This should further be practiced in the measurement of SES. The inconsistency of the relationship between SES and health disparities in the surgical literature has been largely attributed to the variance in the measure of SES. A lack of precise and reliable measures, challenges in collecting individual SES data, and the dynamic nature of SES over an individual's lifetime have all been reported as sources of bias in the measurement of SES.[40] Furthermore, the manner in which SES is coded into databases may offer an incomplete descriptor of socioeconomic vulnerability. Median income, ZIP code of residence, and education level are all metrics used to measure SES, with large variance in association with reported health disparities. The geographic measures used in identifying SES are similarly faulty. ZIP codes were created by the US Postal Service for the purpose of mail delivery but very poorly represent the composition of neighborhoods. More granular geographic information based in Census block or tract level can serve to provide more granular information about patient neighborhoods and social determinants. Furthermore, many of the larger surgical databases do not collect socioeconomic information at the individual level. Comparisons made between population groups and the conclusions drawn should be from data sets with standardized reporting of demographic factors and more representative proxies for SES. Consideration of a more qualitative or prospective research design may also be considered to bypass the limitations posed by the retrospective database studies common to a large body of the surgical disparities literature.

Data Interpretation

Although there are limitations in the databases used to study disparities, there is a plethora of research highlighting health disparities among various marginalized groups.[41–43] However, conclusions drawn from analyses are themselves biased and may be based on faulty preconceptions. Similarly, few go on to study interventions to address disparities at their source. SES is inherently linked to marginalized groups because of long histories of discrimination. For example, black Americans more often live in poverty, have unstable housing, and are concentrated into urban areas largely because of racist housing practices of the 1930s and perpetuated segregation to this day.[44] However, instead of pointing to discrimination as the source of disparities, many studies default to genetic differences as a reason for disparities.[45] Marginalized classifications, including race, are themselves socially and politically constructed and, as such, based on the discrimination imposed on these groups. By highlighting nonmodifiable factors, such as genetics and race, without addressing the modifiable risk factors based in discrimination, researchers risk perpetuating the very disparities they are attempting to address.

OPTIMIZATION OF STUDY DESIGN

First and foremost, health care disparities stem from discrimination based on social designations and constructs. A fundamental limitation of population-based research in thoracic surgery is the lack of infrastructure to comprehensively study health disparities and a lack of adequate understanding on the part of researchers to make informed conclusions from studies. This stems from the aforementioned variances in data sources, data analysis, and importantly, approach to study design. As a result, many of the conclusions and reports of health disparities made in other fields are applied or even inferred in thoracic surgery.

The lack of granular, quality data in thoracic surgery is a major issue for health disparities researchers. From sample size limitations to oversampling, extending into data pooling and use of proxy variables, the heterogeneity of data sources and collection methods poses a major challenge in study methodology. This is in part because of the different registries and lack of standardization across thoracic surgical data sets from which health disparities research draws from. Information management protocols and more standardized national sample data are also needed to identify disparities across major populations. Furthermore, the need for collecting granular data based in social group designations and socioeconomic information is apparent to reduce many measurement errors, but may raise other methodological questions.

Systems-based limitations must also be acknowledged in the thoracic surgery community. Dismal inclusion of marginalized groups is well established, highlighting the need for more effective community outreach and patient-clinician communication strategies, not only to lessen the health disparities gap but also to improve the accuracy of conclusions derived from population-based studies. Patient-centered research and inclusion of representatives of marginalized groups for data collection and interpretation are crucial for drawing robust conclusions (see Rian M. Hasson Charles and colleagues' article "Health Disparities in Recruitment and Enrollment in Research," in this issue).

Overall, it is concerning that there are such lapses in quality data and literature on health disparities in thoracic surgery. It is possible that as providers, thoracic surgeons are not as interested in health disparities research or aware of the entrenched discrimination that leads to them. As mentioned previously, patient participation may also be limited; however, these limitations are present in other fields, which have a relatively established infrastructure for disparities research in comparison to thoracic surgery.[46–48] It may be prudent to adopt existing methodologies until study design strategies for thoracic surgery disparities research mature (**Box 1**). Otherwise, many conclusions in population-based studies in thoracic surgery will continue to rely on missing and limited data, with potential for artificial analysis.

The impact of the SDH at the systems level for surgical research is also not well described as gleaned from the earlier summary of large retrospective databases as the basis for disparities research in thoracic surgery. SES is inherently based in histories of discrimination. Black and brown individuals more often live in poverty because of segregation and preclusion from home ownership.[44] Women are more poorly represented in leadership positions and make less than their male counterparts because of ingrained misogyny. LGBTQ+ individuals are more likely to

> **Box 1**
> **Recommendations for thoracic surgeons to engage in disparities research**
>
> Improved representation of minoritized patients among research subjects.
>
> Improved representation of researchers from minoritized groups or those with subject expertise in study design and interpretation.
>
> Better understanding of discriminatory history underlying health disparities.
>
> Improved granularity of research data to represent minoritized groups and geographic/socioeconomic information.
>
> Greater emphasis on social justice as solution for health care disparities.

experience housing instability because of discrimination and violence against those in this group.[49] These are only a small representation of the vast socioeconomic differences based in social discrimination that underlie SDH. Overall, discrimination leads to marginalization, and researchers identifying these disparities must understand the history of discrimination that leads to these health differences, which are often based in socioeconomic differences themselves. SDH lead to disparities throughout medical and surgical disciplines. This common omission in methodology should compel thoracic surgeons to identify the root social causes of these disparities in order to improve their patients' outcomes.

Much as race, sex, gender, and sexual orientation are social constructions, so too are the discriminatory policies that target these groups.[50] The SDH are inherently tied to these marginalized groups because of preclusion from resources. Physicians become frustrated from lack of ability to address issues around SDH within the health care system, so it is important to realize how policies impact patients. To make actionable change, physicians must advocate for their patients in and out of the hospital. Health equity serves to allocate resources to those for whom they have been precluded for so long; however, we must continue to look forward to social justice where the very inequitable infrastructure that leads to these disparities is reshaped to provide everyone with equal opportunities. Health disparities become apparent in the hospital, but the cause lies in society, so physicians must become aware of the impact of historical policies in shaping health inequity, and prospective policies that can work to deconstruct the discriminatory fabric that leads to disparities.

SUMMARY

The current review offers a summary of current methodological challenges in disparities research in thoracic surgery. The scarcity of high-powered, thorough literature on health disparities in thoracic surgery seems to stem from a lack of quality data. This is not only a result of patient participation but also suggests a lack of interest from researchers in the thoracic surgery community. If thoracic surgeons do not acknowledge the deficiencies and infancy of disparities research methodology, the health disparities gap will struggle to close within the community. In the interim, thoracic surgeons and researchers in thoracic surgery should rely on the infrastructure established by other fields as the framework of health disparities research in thoracic surgery matures because the cause of disparities in all fields lies in social determinants. Similarly, researchers should better understand the historical and political structures in which these disparities are bred to make correct conclusions based on their findings, which can come from diverse research teams. Until then, it is crucial to raise awareness of the complexities and biases in disparities research methodologies, from selecting data sources to final analysis.

CLINICS CARE POINTS

- Researchers in thoracic surgery require education on the sociopolitical roots of health disparities to understand the definitions commonly used in health disparities research.
- The heterogeneity of large clinical registries, from which health disparity outcomes are drawn, must be approached with caution, with a tailored approach for data source selection, as it aligns with the research question being addressed.
- Patient-centered research with focused inclusion of marginalized groups for data collection and interpretation is needed to establish accurate conclusions.
- Community outreach measures directed at patients and thoracic surgery researchers alike are needed to improve the quality of health disparities population studies in thoracic surgery.
- Thoracic surgeons and researchers in the field must appreciate the historical and political structures of health disparities, to make correct conclusions toward health disparities population studies.

DISCLOSURE

This work was partially supported by TUFCCC/HC Regional Comprehensive Cancer Health Disparity Partnership, Award Number U54 CA221704(5) (Contact PIs: Grace X. Ma, PhD and Olorunseun O. Ogunwobi, MD, PhD) from the National Cancer Institute of National Institutes of Health (NCI/NIH) and The American Cancer Society – Pfizer Health Disparities Grant. The content is solely the responsibility of the authors and does not necessarily represent the official views of the funding agencies.

REFERENCES

1. National Center for Health Statistics. Healthy People 2010: Final Review. 2012.
2. Institute of Medicine (US) Committee on Guidance for Designing a National Healthcare Disparities Report, Swift EK, eds. Guidance for the National Healthcare Disparities Report. Washington (DC): National Academies Press (US); 2002.
3. Zimmerman FJ, Anderson NW. Trends in health equity in the United States by race/ethnicity, sex, and income, 1993-2017. JAMA Netw Open 2019. https://doi.org/10.1001/jamanetworkopen.2019.6386.
4. Levine AA, de Jager E, Britt LD. Perspective: identifying and addressing disparities in surgical access. Ann Surg 2020. https://doi.org/10.1097/sla.0000000000003572.
5. Ingram MCE, Calabro K, Polites S, et al. Systematic review of disparities in care and outcomes in pediatric appendectomy. J Surg Res 2020. https://doi.org/10.1016/j.jss.2019.12.018.
6. Bonner SN, Wakam GK, Kwayke G, et al. COVID-19 and racial disparities: moving towards surgical equity. Ann Surg 2020. https://doi.org/10.1097/SLA.0000000000004111.
7. Harper S, Lynch J, Meersman SC, et al. An overview of methods for monitoring social disparities in cancer with an example using trends in lung cancer incidence by area-socioeconomic position and race-ethnicity, 1992-2004. Am J Epidemiol 2008. https://doi.org/10.1093/aje/kwn016.
8. Center for Health Statistics N. Healthy People 2020 leading health indicators. Lead Heal Indic 2030. 2020.
9. Braveman P. What are health disparities and health equity? We need to be clear. Public Health Rep 2014. https://doi.org/10.1177/00333549141291s203.
10. Keppel K, Pamuk E, Lynch J, et al. Methodological issues in measuring health disparities. Vital Health Stat 2 2005;141:1–16.
11. Haider AH, Dankwa-Mullan I, Maragh-Bass AC, et al. Setting a national agenda for surgical disparities research recommendations from the National Institutes of Health and American College of Surgeons summit. JAMA Surg 2016. https://doi.org/10.1001/jamasurg.2016.0014.
12. Cookson R. Inequalities in Health : Concepts, Measures and Ethics, edited by Nir Eyal, Samia A. Hurst, Ole F. Norheim and Dan Wikler. Oxford University Press, 2013, 348 pages. Economics and Philosophy 2015;31(2):312–320.
13. Pronk NP, Kleinman DV, Richmond TS. Healthy People 2030: moving toward equitable health and well-being in the United States. EClinicalMedicine 2021. https://doi.org/10.1016/j.eclinm.2021.100777.
14. Ravi P, Sood A, Schmid M, et al. Racial/ethnic disparities in perioperative outcomes of major procedures: results from the National Surgical Quality Improvement Program. Ann Surg 2015. https://doi.org/10.1097/SLA.0000000000001078.
15. Claflin J, Dimick JB, Campbell DA, et al. Understanding disparities in surgical outcomes for Medicaid beneficiaries. World J Surg 2019. https://doi.org/10.1007/s00268-018-04891-y.
16. Martinez-Meehan D, Abdallah H, Lutfi W, et al. Racial disparity in surgical therapy for thymic malignancies. Chest 2020. https://doi.org/10.1016/j.chest.2020.11.048.
17. Yorio JT, Yan J, Xie Y, et al. Socioeconomic disparities in lung cancer treatment and outcomes persist within a single academic medical center. Clin Lung Cancer 2012. https://doi.org/10.1016/j.cllc.2012.03.002.
18. Chetty R, Hendren N, Katz LF. The effects of exposure to better neighborhoods on children: new evidence from the moving to opportunity experiment. Am Econ Rev 2016;106(4):855–902.
19. Haider AH, Scott VK, Rehman KA, et al. Racial disparities in surgical care and outcomes in the United States: a comprehensive review of patient, provider, and systemic factors. J Am Coll Surg 2013. https://doi.org/10.1016/j.jamcollsurg.2012.11.014.
20. Du XL, Liu CC. Racial/ethnic disparities in socioeconomic status, diagnosis, treatment and survival among Medicare-insured men and women with head and neck cancer. J Health Care Poor Underserved 2010. https://doi.org/10.1353/hpu.0.0331.
21. Kilbourne AM, Switzer G, Hyman K, et al. Advancing health disparities research within the health care system: a conceptual framework. Am J Public Health 2006. https://doi.org/10.2105/AJPH.2005.077628.
22. Ultee KHJ, Tjeertes EKM, Gonçalves FB, et al. The relation between household income and surgical outcome in the Dutch setting of equal access to and provision of healthcare. PLoS One 2018. https://doi.org/10.1371/journal.pone.0191464.
23. Crenshaw KW. Intersectionality, identity politics and violence against women of color. Kvind Køn Forsk 2006. https://doi.org/10.7146/kkf.v0i2-3.28090.

24. Caiola C, Docherty SL, Relf M, et al. Using an intersectional approach to study the impact of social determinants of health for African American mothers living with HIV. ANS Adv Nurs Sci 2014;37(4): 287–98.
25. Winchester DP, Stewart AK, Phillips JL, et al. Editorial: the National Cancer Data Base: past, present, and future. Ann Surg Oncol 2010. https://doi.org/10.1245/s10434-009-0771-3.
26. Gabriel E, Narayanan S, Attwood K, et al. Disparities in major surgery for esophagogastric cancer among hospitals by case volume. J Gastrointest Oncol 2018. https://doi.org/10.21037/jgo.2018.01.18.
27. Dixon JL, Papaconstantinou HT, Hodges B, et al. Redundancy and variability in quality and outcome reporting for cardiac and thoracic surgery. Bayl Univ Med Cent) 2015. https://doi.org/10.1080/08998280.2015.11929173.
28. Servais EL, Towe CW, Brown LM, et al. The Society of Thoracic Surgeons General Thoracic Surgery Database: 2020 update on outcomes and research. Ann Thorac Surg 2020. https://doi.org/10.1016/j.athoracsur.2020.06.006.
29. Shahian DM, Jacobs JP, Edwards FH, et al. The Society of Thoracic Surgeons national database. Heart 2013. https://doi.org/10.1136/heartjnl-2012-303456.
30. National Cancer Institute. Overview of the SEER Program. Available at: http://seer.cancer.gov/about/. 2010. Accessed June 2, 2021.
31. Pasquinelli MM, Kovitz KL, Koshy M, et al. Outcomes from a minority-based lung cancer screening program vs the national lung screening trial. JAMA Oncol 2018. https://doi.org/10.1001/jamaoncol.2018.2823.
32. Martin AN, Hassinger TE, Kozower BD, et al. Disparities in lung cancer screening availability: lessons from Southwest Virginia. Ann Thorac Surg 2019. https://doi.org/10.1016/j.athoracsur.2019.03.003.
33. Lake M, Shusted CS, Juon HS, et al. Black patients referred to a lung cancer screening program experience lower rates of screening and longer time to follow-up. BMC Cancer 2020. https://doi.org/10.1186/s12885-020-06923-0.
34. Han SS, Chow E, Ten Haaf K, et al. Disparities of National Lung Cancer Screening Guidelines in the US population. J Natl Cancer Inst 2020. https://doi.org/10.1093/jnci/djaa013.
35. Steiling K, Loui T, Asokan S, et al. Age, race, and income are associated with lower screening rates at a safety net hospital. Ann Thorac Surg 2020;109(5): 1544–50.
36. Wang GX, Baggett TP, Pandharipande PV, et al. Barriers to lung cancer screening engagement from the patient and provider perspective. Radiology 2019. https://doi.org/10.1148/radiol.2018180212.
37. Rhodes W. Improving disparity research by imputing missing data in health care records. Health Serv Res 2015. https://doi.org/10.1111/1475-6773.12336.
38. Bilheimer LT, Klein RJ. Data and measurement issues in the analysis of health disparities. Health Serv Res 2010. https://doi.org/10.1111/j.1475-6773.2010.01143.x.
39. Lam MB, Raphael K, Mehtsun WT, et al. Changes in racial disparities in mortality after cancer surgery in the US, 2007-2016. JAMA Netw Open 2020. https://doi.org/10.1001/jamanetworkopen.2020.27415.
40. Shavers VL. Measurement of socioeconomic status in health disparities research. J Natl Med Assoc 2007. https://doi.org/10.13016/avw3-9cvx.
41. Du XL, Lin CC, Johnson NJ, et al. Effects of individual-level socioeconomic factors on racial disparities in cancer treatment and survival. Cancer 2011. https://doi.org/10.1002/cncr.25854.
42. Johnson AM, Hines RB, Johnson JA, et al. Treatment and survival disparities in lung cancer: the effect of social environment and place of residence. Lung Cancer 2014. https://doi.org/10.1016/j.lungcan.2014.01.008.
43. Bach PB, Cramer LD, Warren JL, et al. Racial differences in the treatment of early-stage lung cancer. N Engl J Med 1999. https://doi.org/10.1056/nejm199910143411606.
44. Pattillo M. The color of law: a forgotten history of how our government segregated America. Contemp Sociol A J Rev 2018. https://doi.org/10.1177/0094306118792220ll.
45. Jones CC, Mercaldo SF, Blume JD, et al. Racial disparities in lung cancer survival: the contribution of stage, treatment, and ancestry. J Thorac Oncol 2018. https://doi.org/10.1016/j.jtho.2018.05.032.
46. Colon-Otero G, Smallridge RC, Solberg LA, et al. Disparities in participation in cancer clinical trials in the United States: a symptom of a healthcare system in crisis. Cancer 2008. https://doi.org/10.1002/cncr.23201.
47. Gwynn KB, Winter MR, Cabral HJ, et al. Racial disparities in patient activation: evaluating the mediating role of health literacy with path analyses. Patient Educ Couns 2016. https://doi.org/10.1016/j.pec.2015.12.020.
48. Kripalani S, Goggins K, Couey C, et al. Disparities in research participation by level of health literacy. Mayo Clin Proc 2021. https://doi.org/10.1016/j.mayocp.2020.06.058.
49. Fraser B, Pierse N, Chisholm E, et al. LGBTIQ+ homelessness: a review of the literature. Int J Environ Res Public Health 2019. https://doi.org/10.3390/ijerph16152677.
50. Haney-Lopez I. Social construction of race: some observations on illusion, fabrication, and choice. Harvard Civ Rights - Civ Lib Law Rev 1994;29(10): 1–62.

Health Disparities in Recruitment and Enrollment in Research

Rian M. Hasson Charles, MD, MPH, FACS[a], Ernesto Sosa, MSW, MPH[b],
Meghna Patel, BS[b], Loretta Erhunmwunsee, MD[b],*

KEYWORDS

- Thoracic research • Research diversity • Research disparities • Recruitment disparities
- Health disparities • Enrollment disparities • Underrepresented minorities

KEY POINTS

- A lack of representation in thoracic research of racial/ethnic minorities and those of low socioeconomic position exacerbates the disparities that they already experience.
- A lack of racial and socioeconomic diversity in research impedes the ability to advance medical science.
- Several barriers exist that impede diverse research recruitment and enrollment, including, but not limited to, cultural insensitivity, medical mistrust, patient/provider trial unawareness, and provider bias.
- Culturally tailored interventions and research awareness can increase recruitment and enrollment of underrepresented minorities.
- Diversity in research is necessary to increase generalizability of findings, address health disparities, and promote health equity.

INTRODUCTION

There has been considerable progress within thoracic oncology research over the last several decades. We have seen a remarkable refinement of minimally invasive techniques as well as the surge of life-prolonging combination systemic therapy regimens. We have randomized controlled trials that reveal mortality benefit from lung cancer screening and from neoadjuvant and adjuvant systemic therapies. Although lung cancer incidence and mortality rates have subsequently decreased, the benefits of these efforts are not experienced by all groups equally, in part due to the fact that clinical trials specifically, and thoracic research in general, have not included or focused on underrepresented minorities (URM) and those of low

socioeconomic status (SES) at appropriate rates. There are huge disparities in recruitment and enrollment in thoracic research along racial, ethnic, and socioeconomic lines. These disparities lead to inadequate representation in trials, which prevents differential effects among diverse groups from being understood and therefore limits the generalizability of trial results. These race/ethnic and SES-based gaps in research enrollment also contribute to the thoracic-based health care disparities that persist.

Currently, 13% of the US population is African American, 18.5% is Hispanic/Latino, 5.9% Asian, and 1.3% is Native American and Alaska Native.[1] Despite these proportions, only 10% of the landmark National Lung Screening Trial (NLST) participants were non-White and very few participants in

Funded by: NIHHYB. Grant number(s): K12 CA001727/CA/NCI NIH HHS/United States
[a] Dartmouth-Hitchcock Medical Center Geisel School of Medicine at Dartmouth, One Medical Center Drive, Lebanon, NH 03756, USA; [b] City of Hope Comprehensive Cancer Center, 1500 E Duarte Road, Duarte, CA 91010, USA
* Corresponding author.
E-mail address: LorettaE@coh.org

Thorac Surg Clin 32 (2022) 75–82
https://doi.org/10.1016/j.thorsurg.2021.09.012
1547-4127/22/© 2021 Elsevier Inc. All rights reserved.

NLST were of low SES,[2] despite active recruitment.[3,4] In addition, the most cited and practice defining studies in our specialty either give no details to the racial or ethnic breakdown of their cohorts' participants[4-8] or are predominantly White.[9] These cohorts then do not represent the diverse populations in our country who have the highest risk, incidence, and mortality from thoracic cancers. In addition, very few studies describe SES differences among participants.

We must consider that the health care disparities that exist along incidence, risk, and outcome lines may be related to the lack of engagement of minority and low SES communities in thoracic research. Therefore, health equity will not be obtained without a focus on appropriate recruitment of disparate groups. In this chapter, we discuss the importance of enrollment of diverse populations, the barriers to this necessary enrollment, potential facilitators for enrollment, as well as interventions to increase enrollment.

IMPORTANCE OF ENROLLMENT

Differences in health care outcomes among minority and low SES populations remain prevalent. Although many factors contribute to these disparities, a lack of research to better understand these differential health outcomes contributes greatly. In order to use research to address health disparities, it is essential for these studies to include diverse populations. Although the NIH Revitalization Act of 1993 was passed to require the inclusion of minority populations in NIH-funded research, the amount of minority patients enrolled in cancer clinical trials remains low[10] and does not reflect the proportion of minorities that exist in the US population.[11] Participation in oncology research can potentially benefit patients with effective interventions and ultimately improve survival.[12,13] Without equal representation of minorities in oncology research, results are not generalizable across the entire population[14-16] and only certain individuals will benefit. For example, the NLST was monumental in demonstrating how utilization of low-dose computed tomography scans can reduce lung cancer mortality[17]; however, the population sampled was not representative of the entirety of the United States. Participants of the study were 90.8% White, more educated, and younger than the general population. The trial was incredibly successful with high compliance rates and adherence; however, it is unclear if the outcomes would persist in a more diverse patient population or whether barriers might exist. Ultimately, it is imperative to enroll and recruit minority and low SES populations for inclusivity and generalizability in

research in order to directly address current disparities in cancer outcomes.

Underrepresentation of URM and low SES communities in oncology clinical trials mirrors current inequities in the US health care system[14,18]; furthermore, underrepresentation in oncology research may exacerbate existing health disparities. Clinical trials offer access to high-quality health care that can improve survivorship of patients.[14] Without adequate representation, the root causes of disproportionate cancer risk are not accounted for[14] or understood. In addition, cancer disparities cannot be ameliorated without understanding how socioeconomic, cultural, and environmental conditions differ among minority groups and how those factors affect cancer risk, treatment, and survival.[18] Similarly appropriate treatment plans and interventions for minority patients cannot be implemented,[19] which perpetuates the cycle of differential cancer outcomes.

A lack of racial and socioeconomic diversity in research impedes the ability to advance medical science. Information obtained from clinical trials is incredibly important in improving methods of prevention, early diagnosis, and treatment of malignant cancers.[20] Recruitment of minority patients in these trials is essential in bridging the gap between scientific innovation and improving health care delivery and health outcomes for those who are disproportionately affected. Underenrollment of minorities also limits the possibility of conducting subgroup analysis to determine intervention differences among different ethnic origins.[15] Including minority patients in cancer research is crucial to make outcomes generalizable, to make strides toward eliminating health disparities, and to improve understanding of medical science. As such, barriers to recruitment and enrollment into research must be examined and addressed.

BARRIERS TO RECRUITMENT/ENROLLMENT

Several factors contribute to low rates of URM and low SES community participation in cancer research both at an individual and system level. Cultural barriers for both researchers and participants are common obstacles in minority recruitment. For researchers, lack of knowledge on cultural differences among URM can affect research enrollment. Recruitment materials should be culturally and linguistically adapted for the population of interest to effectively communicate the purpose of participation in a culturally sensitive way to patients.[14,21,22] For example, for some culturally diverse populations, the decision-making process involves the patient's family or community; thus, it is important to include families and communities in the conversation about research participation and informed consent. In addition, cultural beliefs of minority patients need to be acknowledged, as they may influence patients' willingness to participate in the research, especially if their beliefs conflict with being enrolled in a clinical trial.[21,22]

A primary cultural barrier to minority recruitment into research trials has been medical mistrust. In one systematic review looking at barriers to recruiting underrepresented populations to cancer clinical trials, mistrust of medical research was the most frequently reported barrier across 65 studies.[23] Minority patients may have negative race-related attitudes and beliefs that stem from racism and discrimination at multiple levels, influencing their decision to take part in research.[14,21,23] The US Public Health Services Syphilis Study at Tuskegee among African Americans and efforts to sterilize Native American women are horrific examples of mistreatment and abuse in medical research of minorities, which could have fostered minority distrust in research participation.[15,21,24,25] Mistrust of the medical community stems from beliefs of purposeful mistreatment, outcomes not benefiting ethnic minorities or their communities, a fear of unintended outcomes or treatment efficacy, and a fear of disclosure of health status and deportation.[21,22,24,26,27] This mistrust and fear accompany the lack of culturally appropriate and sensitive recruitment.

URM and low SES patients also face resource-driven barriers to enrollment. The financial burden of enrollment into cancer research disproportionately affects marginalized patients, as they are more likely to be underinsured and receive care at underresourced hospitals.[14] Among most patients, cost concerns play a large role in study participation decisions.[14,22,26] Furthermore, fear of or actual inadequate insurance coverage for participation in clinical trials is a prevalent barrier to enrollment among several underrepresented groups.[14,22,26] In one study that specifically looked at attitudinal barriers to participation in oncology clinical trials, greater financial burden was associated with more attitudinal barriers to enrollment including discomfort with research or fear of side effects.[26] Other well-established patient-level barriers to enrollment of minority and low SES groups include time constraints and lack of transportation. URM individuals reported having insufficient time to participate in cancer research due to working multiple jobs or working full-time, a lack of childcare, and being the single head of household.[14,21,23,26] These barriers limit patients' ability to follow through with a trial protocol.

Access to research opportunities and awareness of available trials also significantly limit enrollment of minority and low SES populations in cancer research. Many cancer clinical trials are only available in academic settings, which can limit access for minority and low SES patients who receive care in a community-based or underresourced setting.[14,22] In addition, strict eligibility criteria for cancer trials make it difficult for marginalized patients to participate, as they are more likely to present with comorbidities that make them ineligible for trials,[14,23] even if the condition is unrelated to their cancer.[28] More than half of all patients with cancer do not participate in clinical trials because none are available to them. When trials have been available, 21.5% of patients were ineligible.[28] Patients' own lack of awareness of cancer clinical research and their eligibility to participate is also a common barrier that disproportionately affects minority population recruitment.[21–23,26] This further supports the need for bilingual/culturally sensitive informational material and research staff to enhance patient comprehension of the research.

Lastly, provider-driven barriers have been shown to play a significant role in impeding the enrollment of diverse patient populations.[14,22,28] For example, some providers are not aware of the availability or existence of clinical studies for which their patients are eligible.[14,22,29] Provider-driven barriers in minority patient enrollment may result from a lack of support and incentives for providers to participate or from time constraints that limit the opportunity to discuss patient eligibility.[22,28] Provider beliefs that clinical trials lack value for their patients or that discussions focused on clinical trials with minority patients may negatively affect their provider-patient relationship may also lead to low enrollment.[22] Implicit provider biases also deter them from discussing research opportunities with URM patients. Health care professionals may view minorities as less trusting, less likely to adhere to recommended treatments, less likely to comprehend the technicalities of clinical trials, and less compatible with trials.[14,22,26,29] These biases affect the patient-provider relationship, which further deters minority patients from participating in clinical research as well.[14,21,22,30] Despite evidence of these barriers, research that specifically focuses on minority patients is lacking, limiting the information available to fully understand barriers to participation in clinical research for underrepresented groups.[21]

FACILITATORS FOR ENROLLMENT

The most important way to engage underrepresented, underserved, and minority populations in research is to integrate a recruitment of these populations into the study design. Clinical trials should specifically recruit participants who match the demographic make-up of the disease process.[14] Dedicated financial resources and strategic planning dramatically increased participation of underserved populations at specific sites in the NLST.[3] Efforts to increase recruitment should integrate regional factors of patients, health care providers, and community organizations as well as collaboration among these groups.[31-49] Developing these relationships before study protocol development or study start encourages culturally relevant research processes informed by feedback. The National Cancer Institute's (NCI) Minority-Based Community Clinical Oncology Program contributes its success in increasing minority participation in cancer clinical trials to developing relationships with local physicians and cancer advocacy groups, which increased their likelihood of enrolling or referring minority patients to clinical trials.[14] In addition, a biomedical Autism Spectrum Disorder study conducted in Los Angeles showed significant increases in recruitment for Latino families by reaching out to families through an ethnic-specific parent support and advocacy organization.[50] Strategies such as these develop relationships and create trust between participants and researchers.[14,50,51]

Designing trials with effective participation of underrepresented groups requires strategic development of research personnel. Hiring research staff from the community or individuals who reflect community and cultural demographics as part of the research team improves study enrollment.[41] Researchers can establish trust within a community by matching recruiters with participants along ethnic, cultural, and linguistic lines. Strategies using culturally sensitive approaches that build rapport with perspective patients, and obtain provider support, have shown to be the most effective.[52] Integrating diverse staff into research teams can be extremely successful, as potential research participants may view them as more trustworthy based on perceived shared experiences. As an added support, patient navigation programs can offer culturally competent staff for coordination and navigation of the health care and research systems to increase retention.[43,53] Together these methods can be used to put community members in active research roles throughout the research process, creating a framework that helps increase accrual in research studies and adds value to the community.[53]

Similarly, a deliberate strategy to engage the target population will increase participation in clinical trials. Materials adapted to the community of interest in terms of packaging, language, and literacy have all been successful in increasing study enrollment.[27,32] Culturally tailored approaches also allow a space for creativity, by expanding the mediums available for delivering research information. Programs have been able to improve enrollment through diverse delivery methods including television ads from locally recognized news anchors, culturally tailored educational videos, patient-focused scripts for research staff, newsletters, brochures, and personalized stories from previous research participants.[54,55] Lastly, technological components of patient care can be leveraged to enroll populations that are difficult to reach. As electronic medical records (EMR) become integral to our health care system and patient care, they can be used as a reliable means of patient outreach. Using EMR-based methods to enroll patients was shown to have higher recruitment yields and lower costs compared with non-EMR–based methods and significantly increase African American enrollment compared with traditional methods.[56] Educating minority and underrepresented populations about the process and goals of clinical trials is vital to increasing uptake. Benefits gained from participation, at the individual level and the population level, are often not discussed. Research concepts can be hard to understand if patients do not have experience with clinical trials or a fundamental understanding of the research process.[57] The process of enrolling in a clinical trial and responsibilities of participation may be overwhelming, especially in the context of disease processes relevant to thoracic surgery. Potential research participants should understand their rights, including declining participation without compromising their care and withdrawing from participation once enrolled. Candidate participants should also understand that trials are reviewed by Internal Review Boards that include community advocates. Furthermore, participants should know that research personnel must undergo training in ethical research practices. To increase participation of underrepresented populations, investigators must communicate research processes and goals by integrating a culture of education and mutual respect. To address this, Simon and colleagues created a Research Literacy Support tool.[58] The tool was to assist with research education and consisted of a series of 34 cards introducing key informed consent concepts associated with research. The tool was organized into sections that further described basic research information, study-specific information, and research participants' rights in addition to cards that addressed myths and truths. It also notably included multiple prompts to serve as conversation starters to facilitate discussion between study recruiters and research participants.[59] On evaluation of its benefit, participants in phase 3 studies appreciated an increase in their research knowledge following participation. In the final analysis, although knowledge gaps persisted, this tool was found to have the potential to help advance health equity by specifically addressing the communication barriers between participants and researchers that limit minority participation.[58]

At the provider level, discussion of risks and benefits is often lacking, which we have seen in efforts to promote lung cancer screening.[60] Following review of recorded encounters of providers initiating lung cancer screening, quality of shared decision-making was poor and explanation of potential harms of screening was virtually nonexistent. Furthermore, time spent discussing lung cancer screening was minimal, and there was no evidence that decision aids were used.[60] In addition to provider education, some have proposed the use of patient/participant educators, a strategy initially presented by researchers in the Eastern Cooperative Oncology Group, as a means to circumvent provider shortcomings in education abilities[61]; this would entail the use of both participant and patient educators to meet with prospective research participants and educate them regarding the need for research and minority representation. This patient-centered approach may ultimately be the key to appealing to patient interests and ultimately increasing participation.[61]

Recruitment strategies must be sufficiently versatile to address underrepresented populations based on race, ethnicity, gender, orientation, geography, and socioeconomic status as well as those belonging to multiple underrepresented populations. Although previous discussion emphasizes barriers and facilitators based on race, ethnicity, and sociocultural differences, clinical trials must also address the underrepresentation of women. Certain areas of research have traditionally experienced decreased enrollment including cardiovascular care, and certain cancers, and there is marked underrepresentation of women enrolled in cancer clinical trials by the National Cancer Institute.[62] Although certain subgroups of NCI trials have improved female enrollment, sex disparities are still rampant across clinical trials in general, especially for non-NCI–funded trials. Understanding reasons for these disparities and the sex-based reasons for inequities in enrollment are necessary to make gains. In addition, addressing the intersection of racial/ethnic differences with either sex or gender differences[63] or differences in socioeconomic status is needed in order to truly reach equity.

SUMMARY

The lack of proper representation of minority and marginalized groups in thoracic research and clinical trials contributes to the health inequity that remains so pervasive. Our progress within the thoracic field has been limited by our inability to assure that those with the highest risk, incidence, and mortality from thoracic disease are included in trials focused on improving these outcomes. Furthermore, our practice is based on studies with inadequate numbers of the most vulnerable communities, which undoubtedly contributes to the disparities that URM and low SES populations continue to experience.

We must recruit more underrepresented and low SES participants into thoracic research studies and trials if health equity is to be achieved. To improve enrollment and recruitment rates, a multifactorial approach is recommended. Study teams must collaborate with community partners from the start of the study so that there is understanding and buy-in. There should be communication and feedback obtained from advocacy groups and community organizations. We also recommend using culturally and linguistically sensitive staff and multimedia tools to help participants gain both trust and understanding of the research process, investigator responsibilities, benefits, and risks of the study. We must also acknowledge the past sins of science and medicine toward marginalized communities and speak on how our current studies differ. It should also be acknowledged that provider bias impedes recruitment of underrepresented groups and that cultural sensitivity training and diversity, equity, and inclusion education are therefore mandatory. It is important to provide resources to marginalized groups (eg, financial incentives, flexible/weekend appointments, convenient recruitment locations, and other resources), knowing that socioeconomic factors have a strong impact on enrollment. In addition, we must improve access to trials and research opportunities to marginalized groups, and providers in these communities must be educated on the benefits of studies and incentivized and supported so that they are able to make time to discuss these treatment options with their patients. Integration of technology including social media platforms and electronic medical records can increase access to education and opportunity regarding active studies for both patients and providers. Lastly, funding and support should be provided to assure that studies are compliant with URM and low SES participant recruitment efforts.

In short, until we have appropriate representation of URM and marginalized groups in trials, we will continue to provide subpar care to everyone. Quality care is predicated on assuring that the most vulnerable groups are considered, understood, and their care elevated. We miss out on full discovery if those with the largest barriers, the most aggressive disease, and the worst outcomes are excluded from study. Focused attention on the aforementioned recommendations by every study investigator and team member should get us closer to improved study representation, which will be a significant step toward decreasing health disparities and achieving health equity.

DISCLOSURE

The authors declare no potential conflicts of interest.

REFERENCES

1. United States Census Bureau. US census bureau July 1 2019 estimates 2019. Available at: https://www.census.gov/quickfacts/fact/table/US/PST045219. Accessed April 12, 2021.
2. Aberle DR, Adams AM, Berg CD, et al. Baseline characteristics of participants in the randomized national lung screening trial. J Natl Cancer Inst 2010; 102(23):1771–9.
3. Duda C, Mahon I, Chen MH, et al. Impact and costs of targeted recruitment of minorities to the National Lung Screening Trial. Clin Trials 2011;8(2):214–23.
4. Arriagada R, Bergman B, Dunant A, et al. Cisplatin-based adjuvant chemotherapy in patients with completely resected non-small-cell lung cancer. N Engl J Med 2004;350(4):351–60.
5. van Hagen P, Hulshof MCCM, van Lanschot JJB, et al. Preoperative chemoradiotherapy for esophageal or junctional cancer. N Engl J Med 2012; 366(22):2074–84.
6. Douillard JY, Rosell R, De Lena M, et al. Adjuvant vinorelbine plus cisplatin versus observation in patients with completely resected stage IB-IIIA non-small-cell lung cancer (Adjuvant Navelbine International Trialist Association [ANITA]): a randomised controlled trial. Lancet Oncol 2006;7(9):719–27.
7. Ginsberg RJ, Rubinstein LV. Randomized trial of lobectomy versus limited resection for T1 N0 non-small cell lung cancer. Lung Cancer Study Group. Ann Thorac Surg 1995;60(3):615–22 [discussion 613–22].
8. Rosell R, Gomez-Codina J, Camps C, et al. A randomized trial comparing preoperative chemotherapy plus surgery with surgery alone in patients with non-small-cell lung cancer. N Engl J Med 1994;330(3):153–8.
9. Albain KS, Rusch VW, Crowley JJ, et al. Concurrent cisplatin/etoposide plus chest radiotherapy followed by surgery for stages IIIA (N2) and IIIB non-small-cell lung cancer: mature results of Southwest Oncology Group phase II study 8805. J Clin Oncol 1995;13(8):1880–92.
10. Chen MS Jr, Lara PN, Dang JHT, et al. Twenty years post-NIH Revitalization Act: enhancing minority participation in clinical trials (EMPaCT): laying the groundwork for improving minority clinical trial accrual: renewing the case for enhancing minority participation in cancer clinical trials. Cancer 2014; 120(Suppl 7):1091–6.
11. Fisher JA, Kalbaugh CA. Challenging assumptions about minority participation in US clinical research. Am J Public Health 2011;101(12):2217–22.
12. Chow CJ, Habermann EB, Abraham A, et al. Does enrollment in cancer trials improve survival? J Am Coll Surg 2013;216(4):774–81.
13. Diehl KM, Green EM, Weinberg A, et al. Features associated with successful recruitment of diverse patients onto cancer clinical trials: report from the American College of Surgeons Oncology Group. Ann Surg Oncol 2011;18(13):3544–50.
14. Hamel LM, Penner LA, Albrecht TL, et al. Barriers to clinical trial enrollment in racial and ethnic minority patients with cancer. Cancer Control 2016;23(4): 327–37.
15. Hussain-Gambles M, Atkin K, Leese B. Why ethnic minority groups are under-represented in clinical trials: a review of the literature. Health Soc Care Community 2004;12(5):382–8.
16. Zullig LL, Fortune-Britt AG, Rao S, et al. Enrollment and racial disparities in cancer treatment clinical trials in North Carolina. N C Med J 2016;77(1):52–8.
17. Aberle DR, Berg CD, Black WC, et al. The National Lung Screening Trial: overview and study design. Radiology 2011;258(1):243–53.
18. Newman LA, Roff NK, Weinberg AD. Cancer clinical trials accrual: missed opportunities to address disparities and missed opportunities to improve outcomes for all. Ann Surg Oncol 2008;15(7):1818–9.
19. Nazha B, Mishra M, Pentz R, et al. Enrollment of racial minorities in clinical trials: old problem assumes new urgency in the age of immunotherapy. Am Soc Clin Oncol Educ Book 2019;39:3–10.
20. Langford AT, Resnicow K, Dimond EP, et al. Racial/ethnic differences in clinical trial enrollment, refusal rates, ineligibility, and reasons for decline among patients at sites in the National Cancer Institute's Community Cancer Centers Program. Cancer 2014;120(6):877–84.
21. George S, Duran N, Norris K. A systematic review of barriers and facilitators to minority research participation among African Americans, Latinos, Asian

Americans, and Pacific Islanders. Am J Public Health 2014;104(2):e16–31.

22. Salman A, Nguyen C, Lee Y-H, et al. A review of barriers to minorities' participation in cancer clinical trials: implications for future cancer research. J Immigrant Minor Health 2016;18(2):447–53.

23. Ford JG, Howerton MW, Lai GY, et al. Barriers to recruiting underrepresented populations to cancer clinical trials: a systematic review. Cancer 2008; 112(2):228–42.

24. Corbie-Smith G, Moody-Ayers S, Thrasher AD. Closing the circle between minority inclusion in research and health disparities. Arch Intern Med 2004; 164(13):1362–4.

25. Trantham LC, Carpenter WR, DiMartino LD, et al. Perceptions of cancer clinical research among African American Men in North Carolina. J Natl Med Assoc 2015;107(1):33–41.

26. Manne S, Kashy D, Albrecht T, et al. Attitudinal barriers to participation in oncology clinical trials: factor analysis and correlates of barriers. Eur J Cancer Care 2015;24(1):28–38.

27. Schmotzer GL. Barriers and facilitators to participation of minorities in clinical trials. Ethn Dis 2012; 22(2):226–30.

28. Unger JM, Vaidya R, Hershman DL, et al. Systematic review and meta-analysis of the magnitude of structural, clinical, and physician and patient barriers to cancer clinical trial participation. J Natl Cancer Inst 2019;111(3):245–55.

29. Howerton MW, Gibbons MC, Baffi CR, et al. Provider roles in the recruitment of underrepresented populations to cancer clinical trials. Cancer 2007;109(3): 465–76.

30. Survival of patients with stage i lung cancer detected on CT screening. N Engl J Med 2006; 355(17):1763–71.

31. Andreae SJ, Halanych JH, Cherrington A, et al. Recruitment of a rural, southern, predominantly African-American population into a diabetes self-management trial. Contemp Clin Trials 2012;33(3): 499–506.

32. Bailey JM, Bieniasz ME, Kmak D, et al. Recruitment and retention of economically underserved women to a cervical cancer prevention trial. Appl Nurs Res 2004;17(1):55–60.

33. Baquet CR. A model for bidirectional community-academic engagement (CAE): overview of partnered research, capacity enhancement, systems transformation, and public trust in research. J Health Care Poor Underserved 2012;23(4): 1806–24.

34. Baquet CR, Henderson K, Commiskey P, et al. Clinical trials: the art of enrollment. Semin Oncol Nurs 2008;24(4):262–9.

35. Burns D, Soward AC, Skelly AH, et al. Effective recruitment and retention strategies for older members of rural minorities. Diabetes Educ 2008; 34(6):1045–52.

36. Eakin EG, Bull SS, Riley K, et al. Recruitment and retention of Latinos in a primary care-based physical activity and diet trial: The Resources for Health study. Health Educ Res 2007;22(3):361–71.

37. Ellis SD, Bertoni AG, Bonds DE, et al. Value of recruitment strategies used in a primary care practice-based trial. Contemp Clin Trials 2007;28(3):258–67.

38. Ezeugwu CO, Laird A, Mullins CD, et al. Lessons learned from community-based minority health care serving system participation in an NIH clinical trial. J Natl Med Assoc 2011;103(9–10):839–44.

39. Guadagnolo BA, Petereit DG, Helbig P, et al. Involving American Indians and medically underserved rural populations in cancer clinical trials. Clin Trials 2009;6(6):610–7.

40. Hays J, Hunt JR, Hubbell FA, et al. The Women's Health Initiative recruitment methods and results. Ann Epidemiol 2003;13(9 Suppl):S18–77.

41. Holmes DR, Major J, Lyonga DE, et al. Increasing minority patient participation in cancer clinical trials using oncology nurse navigation. Am J Surg 2012; 203(4):415–22.

42. Lora CM, Ricardo AC, Brecklin CS, et al. Recruitment of Hispanics into an observational study of chronic kidney disease: the Hispanic Chronic Renal Insufficiency Cohort Study experience. Contemp Clin Trials 2012;33(6):1238–44.

43. McCaskill-Stevens W, Pinto H, Marcus AC, et al. Recruiting minority cancer patients into cancer clinical trials: a pilot project involving the Eastern Cooperative Oncology Group and the National Medical Association. J Clin Oncol 1999;17(3):1029–39.

44. McCaskill-Stevens W, Wilson JW, Cook ED, et al. National Surgical Adjuvant Breast and Bowel Project Study of Tamoxifen and Raloxifene trial: advancing the science of recruitment and breast cancer risk assessment in minority communities. Clin Trials 2013;10(2):280–91.

45. Michaels M, Weiss ES, Guidry JA, et al. The promise of community-based advocacy and education efforts for increasing cancer clinical trials accrual. J Cancer Educ 2012;27(1):67–74.

46. Rosal MC, White MJ, Borg A, et al. Translational research at community health centers: challenges and successes in recruiting and retaining low-income Latino patients with type 2 diabetes into a randomized clinical trial. Diabetes Educ 2010; 36(5):733–49.

47. Vicini F, Nancarrow-Tull J, Shah C, et al. Increasing accrual in cancer clinical trials with a focus on minority enrollment: The William Beaumont Hospital Community Clinical Oncology Program Experience. Cancer 2011;117(20):4764–71.

48. Wiemann CM, Chacko MR, Tucker JC, et al. Enhancing recruitment and retention of minority

young women in community-based clinical research. J Pediatr Adolesc Gynecol 2005;18(6): 403–7.

49. Wisdom K, Neighbors K, Williams VH, et al. Recruitment of African Americans with type 2 diabetes to a randomized controlled trial using three sources. Ethn Health 2002;7(4):267–78.

50. Zamora I, Williams ME, Higareda M, et al. Brief report: recruitment and retention of minority children for autism research. J Autism Dev Disord 2016; 46(2):698–703.

51. Reidy MC, Orpinas P, Davis M. Successful recruitment and retention of Latino study participants. Health Promot Pract 2012;13(6):779–87.

52. Jaurretche M, Levy M, Castel AD, et al. Factors influencing successful recruitment of racial and ethnic minority patients for an observational HIV cohort study in Washington, DC. J Racial Ethn Health Disparities 2021. [Epub ahead of print].

53. Greiner KA, Friedman DB, Adams SA, et al. Effective recruitment strategies and community-based participatory research: community networks program centers' recruitment in cancer prevention studies. Cancer Epidemiol Biomarkers Prev 2014;23(3): 416–23.

54. Vuong I, Wright J, Nolan MB, et al. Overcoming barriers: evidence-based strategies to increase enrollment of underrepresented populations in cancer therapeutic clinical trials—a narrative review. J Cancer Educ 2020;35(5):841–9.

55. Robinson BN, Newman AF, Tefera E, et al. Video intervention increases participation of black breast cancer patients in therapeutic trials. NPJ Breast Cancer 2017;3(1):36.

56. Miller HN, Charleston J, Wu B, et al. Use of electronic recruitment methods in a clinical trial of adults with gout. Clin Trials 2020;18(1):92–103.

57. Echeverri M, Anderson D, Nápoles AM, et al. Cancer health literacy and willingness to participate in cancer research and donate bio-specimens. Int J Environ Res Public Health 2018;15(10):2091.

58. Simon MA, Haring R, Rodriguez EM, et al. Improving research literacy in diverse minority populations with a novel communication tool. J Cancer Educ 2019; 34(6):1120–9.

59. Torres S, de la Riva EE, Tom LS, et al. The development of a communication tool to facilitate the cancer trial recruitment process and increase research literacy among underrepresented populations. J Cancer Educ 2015;30(4):792–8.

60. Brenner AT, Malo TL, Margolis M, et al. Evaluating shared decision making for lung cancer screening. JAMA Intern Med 2018;178(10):1311–6.

61. Fong S, Tan A, Czupryn J, et al. Patient-centred education: how do learners' perceptions change as they experience clinical training? Adv Health Sci Educ Theor Pract 2019;24(1):15–32.

62. Murthy VH, Krumholz HM, Gross CP. Participation in cancer clinical trials: race-, sex-, and age-based disparities. JAMA 2004;291(22):2720–6.

63. Streed CG Jr, Lunn MR, Siegel J, et al. Meeting the patient care, education, and research missions: academic medical centers must comprehensively address sexual and gender minority health. Acad Med 2021;96(6):822–7.

Social Disparities in Thoracic Surgery Database Research: Implications and Impact

Kyle G. Mitchell, MD, MSc, Ian C. Bostock, MD, MSc, Mara B. Antonoff, MD*

KEYWORDS

- Thoracic surgery • Database research • Informatics • Health care disparities • Big data
- Non–small cell lung cancer • Esophageal cancer • Mesothelioma

KEY POINTS

- A growing body of literature has documented wide socioeconomic disparities in patient access to and outcomes following surgical care in a variety of clinical settings.
- Large administrative and population-level databases afford opportunities to investigate the presence and extent of social disparities in thoracic surgical patients.
- Structural factors contributing to overrepresentation or underrepresentation of certain sociodemographic populations within these databases exist, which potentially limit the ability to draw reliable conclusions from studies using these data sets.
- Accruing evidence of variation in the bimolecular contexture of thoracic malignancies that differs according to sex and racial/ethnic background supports similar caution when performing studies that rely on large tissue repositories and databanks.

INTRODUCTION

A greater understanding of social disparities in health care promises an ability to establish large-scale interventions that could improve access to and delivery of health care resources to vulnerable socioeconomic and demographic groups. There have been myriad reports throughout the literature describing a wide breadth of socioeconomic disparities in access to care and post-treatment outcomes in a range of settings.[1]

Systematic clinical database research originated as a means of studying health care delivery with the aim of improving the quality of care in the general population. Large databases have been constructed that capture large cohorts by statistical sampling or collection of administrative billing and/or claims data, collection of patient-related data within select health care systems (eg, Department of Veterans Affairs system), and by voluntary institution-level contributions to quality improvement initiatives.[2–10] As these databases have developed and their data gathering mechanisms improved over time, investigators' ability to perform population-level studies using these resources has become more granular and reliable. There are clear limitations, however, in these data, which limit the ability to capture particular patient socioeconomic and demographic data in sufficient detail to fully elucidate their influence on health outcomes of interest. These important confounding variables take an even more complex role in the interpretation of studies relying on analyses of publicly available biomolecular and genomic data sets (eg, The Cancer Genome Atlas [TCGA]).[11–14]

This article presents a review of the available clinical databases used most frequently in large-scale population-level investigation in thoracic surgery, explores the current evidence generated by analyses of these databases that attests to social disparities in the treatment of patients with

Department of Thoracic and Cardiovascular Surgery, University of Texas MD Anderson Cancer Center, 1515 Holcombe Boulevard, Unit 1489, Houston, TX 77030, USA
* Corresponding author.
E-mail address: mbantonoff@mdanderson.org

Thorac Surg Clin 32 (2022) 83–90
https://doi.org/10.1016/j.thorsurg.2021.09.007
1547-4127/22/© 2021 Elsevier Inc. All rights reserved.

thoracic malignancies, and examines distinct opportunities for improvement of the quality and inclusiveness of clinical databases afforded by novel big data analytical methods.

CURRENT EVIDENCE
Available Databases and Their Application to Identify Disparities in Thoracic Surgical Care

Large clinical databases capture patients treated at multiple institutions with unified data collection and quality control mechanisms to provide a valuable lens via which structural disparities in access to and outcomes following care may be examined. As such, retrospective analyses of these large databases have been used to identify and to highlight these disparities. A summary of available data sets and examples of their use to identify disparities that warrant finer dissection in future investigations are discussed.

The Society of Thoracic Surgeons (STS) General Thoracic Surgery Database (GTSD) collects clinicopathologic, treatment, and perioperative outcome data on patients undergoing thoracic surgical operations at participating centers.[3,4] Although a review of the literature suggests a relative paucity of disparities analyses using the GTSD compared with other large data sets, it has been used to identify sex-related differences in 30-day postoperative mortality following lung cancer resection.[15] Other work has identified racial and ethnic differences in rates of postoperative atrial fibrillation following pulmonary resection[16] and in disease stage at the time of resection[17] in non–small cell lung cancer (NSCLC) patients. Similarly, among patients undergoing esophagectomy for esophageal cancer, race was found to be associated with an increased odds of major postoperative morbidity.[18] Although the GTSD does not capture outcomes outside the perioperative period, prior demonstration of the ability of STS databases linkage with Medicare data[19,20] and other administrative databases[21] affords an opportunity to understand the relationships between patient socioeconomic and demographic factors and long-term survival outcomes in this patient cohort.

The National Cancer Database (NCDB) is a repository of clinicopathologic, treatment, and outcome data on patients with cancer who are diagnosed and/or treated at a participating center; as such, it is estimated to capture 70% of incident cancer cases in United States.[2] The NCDB has been used to identify racial variation in receipt of surgery among patients with esophageal cancer,[22] sex disparities in the utilization of surgical therapy and chemotherapy in patients with malignant

pleural mesothelioma,[23] and racial and ethnic variation in receipt of cancer-directed therapy among patients with stage III NSCLC.[24]

A variety of other administrative, quality improvement, and population-level data sets are available for analysis, and each is associated with its own distinct profile of merits and disadvantages. Some, like Medicare claims data[5] and the Veterans Affairs Surgical Quality Improvement Program (VASQIP) data set[6] have broad capture of the underlying patient/beneficiary population. Others, like the National Inpatient Sample[7]; the National Surgical Quality Improvement Program[8]; and the Surveillance, Epidemiology, and End Results (SEER) database,[9] are compiled by hospital-level or population-level sampling methods that are designed to have a high degree of representativeness of relevant patient (socioeconomic and demographic) and health care setting characteristics. In addition, several data sets may be linked to permit longitudinal analysis of patient outcomes and to identify cancer-related data (VASQIP and the Veterans Affairs Central Cancer Registry[6]; SEER-Medicare[5]).

Representativeness and Limitations of Available Clinical Databases

Notwithstanding the utility of large clinical databases in investigation of health care disparities, the representativeness of the patient cohorts captured by these databases warrants close inspection.

Although the NCDB captures a large proportion of incident cancer cases, contribution to the database is voluntary, and only 30% of hospitals in the country participate.[2] As such, there are well-attested disparities in terms of center representation that must be accounted for when interpreting results of analyses of the NCDB. In comparison to data from the US Cancer Statistics registry, the NCDB was noted to have wide variation in case coverage according to geographic location, patient age, sex, racial and ethnic background, and cancer site.[25] These differences in patient demographic composition of clinical databases can have a meaningful impact on results and conclusions according to which database is analyzed: simultaneous analysis of SEER-Medicare and NCDB databases identified differing degrees of delay from diagnosis to resection of breast cancer among several demographic subgroups.[26]

Participation in the STS GTSD similarly is voluntary and has been shown to have low—although increasing—penetrance at the patient and institution levels that is notably lower than that of the STS Adult Cardiac Surgery Database.[3,27,28] As a consequence, data within the GTSD reflects structural characteristics of the institutions and sites that contribute, including a willingness to pay the participation fee, a possible greater degree of surgeon specialization, and acceptance of the use of the GTSD for public outcome reporting.[27]

In addition, idiosyncratic characteristics of the populations comprising administrative and population-level databases must be considered (Table 1). By definition, the Medicare claims data set only captures data for older adults.[5] In contrast, the Military Health System Data Repository of TRICARE claims data set may be more representative of patients under 64 years old, although racial and ethnic data frequently are missing.[10]

Finally, although large administrative and population-level databases are characterized by the benefit of large sample sizes, they may lack sufficient granularity to dissect crucial components adequately and thoroughly, driving disparities in health care access and outcomes. As a representative example, patient income levels and educational attainment are analyzed by the NCDB at the level of zip code and categorized according to quartile.[2] Depending on the data set used, analyses incorporating patient comorbidities, treatment-specific data, and long-term outcomes may be limited or impossible. Novel approaches to analysis of larger institutional and health care system databases that may be used to improve database granularity in large patient cohorts are discussed.

Opportunities Generated by Novel Approaches to Big Data

Novel data processing and analytical tools, including natural language processing and optical character recognition, are being refined to exploit the explosion of health care–related patient data generated by electronic medical records and personal smart devices.[29] Natural language processing allows for structured searches of unstructured data fields to identify terms and keywords of interest. This process allows for scanning large volumes of patient data within electronic medical records and for abstraction of data points and variables of interest for consolidation into more structured databases. More sophisticated approaches allow users to further refine search results based on the relationship between search terms and surrounding text. Optical character recognition may be used to augment preexisting electronic health information by converting scanned documents into digital text that then may be searched, compiled into research databases, and analyzed. The authors' group[29–33] and others[34] previously

have demonstrated the feasibility and utility of use of these analytical tools to facilitate investigative efforts by compiling patient cohorts of interest and by defining key exposure and outcome variables. It is the authors' view that these tools offer an opportunity to broaden the scope of current disparities research in the following ways: first, they permit analysis of large cohorts of patients by scanning large volumes of electronic health information; second, by doing so, they enable identification of rare exposures or outcomes that would otherwise be prohibitively labor-intensive to identify; and third, they allow for abstraction and identification of more granular patient demographic, treatment, and outcome variables from individual hospital, regional, or health care system records than are available in current large, population-level, or administrative databases.

Insight into Clinical Trial Enrollment Disparities Gleaned from Analysis of Trial-related Metadata

The randomized controlled trial (RCT), along with systematic reviews of RCTs, constitutes the highest level of clinical evidence for interventional studies.[35] The National Institutes of Health established ClinicalTrials.gov as a publicly available trial registry with the aim of improving transparency in the conduct and reporting of clinical trials.[36] Because prior trial registration frequently is a prerequisite for publication, ClinicalTrials.gov serves as a rich and up-to-date repository of trial-related metadata that investigators may harness to identify disparities in clinical trial enrollment.

Examination of 302 cancer-related phase 3 RCTs demonstrated a younger median patient age in participants in RCTs than the disease site–specific median age in the SEER database; this difference was most pronounced among industry-sponsored trials and in those restricted to a specific biomolecular or mutational profile.[37] Of the disease sites examined (breast, colorectal, lung, and prostate), patients with lung cancer had the greatest age discrepancy between RCT enrollees and those reported in SEER registry (mean difference in median age −8.98 years, standard error 0.35 years). Although this analysis identified a trend of widening age disparities with time,[37] another somewhat paradoxically found a reduced incidence of explicit age-related exclusion criteria.[38] Other analyses have identified underrepresentation of women[39] and racial and ethnic minorities[40,41] in cancer-related clinical trials and have proved the feasibility of such analyses of RCT metadata using ClinicalTrials.gov.

Table 1
Large clinical databases and key considerations regarding inherent limitations that are relevant to disparities research

Database	Key Considerations
NCDB	Wide variation in case coverage according to geographic location of participating centers and patient socioeconomic/demographic characteristics
STS GTSD	Limited to short-term postoperative outcomes Low penetrance at institution and individual patient/case levels
National Surgical Quality Improvement Program	Limited to short-term postoperative outcomes Hospital-level sampling
SEER	Population-based sampling Lacks granular treatment-related data
VASQIP	Only captures patients treated at Veterans Affairs facilities
Military Health System Data Repository of Tricare	Incomplete racial and ethnic data
Medicare claims database	Only captures patients enrolled on Medicare
National Inpatient Sample	Administrative database Limited clinical information aside from procedure and diagnosis codes

Implications for Biomolecular Research

One of the most dramatic recent successes in the management of patients with NSCLC has been the application of immune checkpoint inhibitor[42,43] and targeted therapies[44] in patients with metastatic and resectable NSCLC. The clinical expansion of the use of these novel therapies has been paralleled by an increasingly nuanced understanding of biomolecular events underpinning oncogenesis, tumor progression, and evasion of the host immune system.[42]

TCGA hosts multi-omics (transcriptomic, genomic, and proteomic) data for a variety of cancers—including NSCLC,[11,14] malignant pleural mesothelioma,[12] and esophageal cancer[45]—and has proved to be an invaluable resource for basic and translational investigations. Despite their rich biomolecular data, the data sets are annotated with limited clinical information, some of which suggests underrepresentation or overrepresentation of demographic subgroups. An inspection of demographic information provided in the index reports of the lung adenocarcinoma (LUAD)[14] and lung squamous cell carcinoma (LUSC)[11] data sets reveals discrepancies in the distribution of sex between the data sets (LUAD, 43.9% men; LUSC, 73.6% men). There exists evidence to suggest that this varying sex distribution could be biologically relevant: an immunohistochemical analysis of 146 patients who underwent resection of stage I to stage III LUAD identified higher intratumoral densities of T lymphocytes and macrophages in women than in men; the finding of increased cytotoxic T-cell infiltration in women was replicated using analysis of gene expression signatures in the TCGA cohort.[46]

In addition, immunogenomic profiling of NSCLCs has identified distinct biomolecular profiles according to patient ethnic and racial background. Profiling of tumors from African American NSCLC patients have identified higher rates of oncogenic mutations (STK11/LKB1 and RB1,[47] PTPRT, and JAK2[48]) and distinct transcriptomic profiles[49,50] compared with patients of European descent as well as the presence of mutations not identified within the TCGA database.[51] Similarly, analysis of the Lung Cancer Mutation Consortium 1 database (composed of 1007 patients) revealed wide variance in the presence of driver mutations among patients of different racial and ethnic backgrounds.[52] In contrast, a study of 509 tumors demonstrated no differences in prevalence of mutations in known oncogenic drivers according to ancestry,[53] and others have come to conflicting conclusions regarding tumor mutational burden and the frequency of targetable mutations.[54]

Although the relationship between patient ethnic and racial background and biomolecular tumor features in NSCLC remains incompletely defined, the aforementioned evidence is of sufficient strength to warrant consideration of patient demographics when constructing, analyzing, and interpreting results from biomolecular tumor databases.

Relevance of Disparities in Patient-reported Outcomes Analyses

Consideration of the impact of thoracic surgical interventions on patient quality of life now is recognized as a priority. Analysis and reporting of patient-reported outcomes (PROs) have become increasingly frequent in oncology trials[55]; as a consequence, construction of PRO databases proves to have an impact on the conduct of retrospective, prospective observational, and prospective interventional studies.

A survey of 175 patients who previously had undergone surgical resection of stage I NSCLC identified differences in patient preferences regarding participation in a structured exercise program, receipt of advice regarding physical activity from physicians versus other health care providers, and type and location of exercise that varied according to patient sex, educational attainment, and reported income.[56] Similarly, investigators have identified differential reporting of a validated stress measure among breast cancer patients[57] and disparate rates of completion of PRO questionnaires and preferred contact methods among patients with urologic cancers[58] that varied according to racial and ethnic background. Critically, an analysis of the ClinicalTrials.gov database demonstrated that 68.0% of oncology randomized trials that used a PRO as a primary endpoint did not validate PRO questionnaires in languages other than English.[59]

As PROs gain increasing relevance as primary, coprimary, and/or secondary outcomes in ongoing and future studies, it will be critical to acknowledge that patient perspectives clearly vary according to socioeconomic and demographic characteristics. Additionally, the influence of these demographic characteristics on patient preferences conceivably could vary temporally throughout a given patient's treatment course. Further work is needed to ensure that socioeconomic and demographic factors are appropriately considered when constructing, validating, and applying PRO assessments in future studies.

DISCUSSION

Health services research and large database investigations have had a substantial impact on clinical practice, improved the ability to track clinical outcomes, and prompted the implementation of quality improvement initiatives. Nonetheless, the

interpretation of conclusions from large database studies, the ability to establish causal links between exposures and outcomes of interest, and the identification of a source for discordant outcomes in underserved populations may be hindered by the nature of the data available from these resources. Investigations of the relationship between socioeconomic and demographic patient characteristics and clinical outcomes in thoracic surgical patients are not exempt from these limitations.

This review highlights examples of investigations leveraging large databases and novel analytical approaches to highlight disparate access to care and discordant outcomes following the treatment of thoracic malignancies. Work must be undertaken to improve representation of all patient subgroups in research databases, to include a varied cohort of hospitals and health care systems, and to deploy novel data gathering techniques to leverage the rapid expansion of available big data ecosystems. Such interventions may help bridge the gap in these settings and ultimately enhance clinical care for underserved patient populations.

SUMMARY

Large clinical databases offer several advantages in population-level analyses of social health care disparities in thoracic surgical patients. Unique characteristics of the underlying patient sample or population comprising each database must be considered carefully when performing and interpreting analyses utilizing these resources. Future work to understand and to improve the representativeness of these data sets is warranted to enhance their ability to have an impact on current and future clinical practice.

CLINICS CARE POINTS

- Access to health care resources, receipt of guideline-concordant care, and outcomes following care among thoracic surgical patients are marked by variation according to patient socioeconomic and demographic factors.
- Large clinical databases permit identification of these disparities and investigation of underlying causes.

- The representativeness of each individual database must be assessed carefully when interpreting data and study results.
- Clear delineation of and identification of strategies to alleviate structural factors contributing to overrepresentation and underrepresentation of patient subgroups are needed to bolster and to increase inclusivity within these database resources.
- Application of results of database research must consider carefully whether a given patient's characteristics are well represented in the database patient sample and, if dissimilar, should be considered with caution.

DISCLOSURE

The authors have nothing to disclose.

REFERENCES

1. Ward E, Jemal A, Cokkinides V, et al. Cancer disparities by race/ethnicity and Socioeconomic Status. CA Cancer J Clin 2004;54(2):78–93.
2. Boffa DJ, Rosen JE, Mallin K, et al. Using the national cancer database for outcomes research: a review. JAMA Oncol 2017;3(12):1722–8.
3. Seder CW, Magee MJ, Broderick SR, et al. The society of thoracic surgeons general thoracic surgery database 2019 update on outcomes and quality. Ann Thorac Surg 2019;107(5):1302–6.
4. Farjah F, Kaji AH, Chu D. Practical guide to surgical data sets: society of thoracic surgeons (STS) national database. JAMA Surg 2018;153(10):955–6.
5. Ghaferi AA, Dimick JB. Practical guide to surgical data sets: Medicare claims data. JAMA Surg 2018; 153(7):677–8.
6. Massarweh NN, Kaji AH, Itani KMF. Practical guide to surgical data sets: veterans affairs surgical quality improvement program (VASQIP). JAMA Surg 2018; 153(8):768–9.
7. Stulberg JJ, Haut ER. Practical guide to surgical data sets: healthcare cost and utilization project national inpatient sample (NIS). JAMA Surg 2018; 153(6):586–7.
8. Raval MV, Pawlik TM. Practical guide to surgical data sets: national surgical quality improvement program (NSQIP) and pediatric NSQIP. JAMA Surg 2018;153(8):764–5.
9. Doll KM, Rademaker A, Sosa JA. Practical guide to surgical data sets: surveillance, epidemiology, and end results (SEER) database. JAMA Surg 2018; 153(6):588–9.
10. Schoenfeld AJ, Kaji AH, Haider AH. Practical guide to surgical data sets: military health system tricare encounter data. JAMA Surg 2018;153(7):679–80.
11. Hammerman PS, Lawrence MS, Voet D, et al. Comprehensive genomic characterization of squamous cell lung cancers. Nature 2012;489(7417): 519–25.
12. Hmeljak J, Sanchez-Vega F, Hoadley KA, et al. Integrative molecular characterization of malignant pleural mesothelioma. Cancer Discov 2018;8(12): 1548–65.
13. Kargl J, Busch SE, Yang GHY, et al. Neutrophils dominate the immune cell composition in non-small cell lung cancer. Nat Commun 2017;8:14381.
14. Collisson EA, Campbell JD, Brooks AN, et al. Comprehensive molecular profiling of lung adenocarcinoma. Nature 2014;511(7511):543–50.
15. Tong BC, Kosinski AS, Burfeind WR Jr, et al. Sex differences in early outcomes after lung cancer resection: analysis of the Society of Thoracic Surgeons General Thoracic Database. J Thorac Cardiovasc Surg 2014;148(1):13–8.
16. Onaitis M, D'Amico T, Zhao Y, et al. Risk factors for atrial fibrillation after lung cancer surgery: analysis of the Society of Thoracic Surgeons general thoracic surgery database. Ann Thorac Surg 2010;90(2): 368–74.
17. Weksler B, Kosinski AS, Burfeind WR, et al. Racial and ethnic differences in lung cancer surgical stage: an STS database study. Thorac Cardiovasc Surg 2015;63(7):538–43.
18. Wright CD, Kucharczuk JC, O'Brien SM, et al. Predictors of major morbidity and mortality after esophagectomy for esophageal cancer: a Society of Thoracic Surgeons General Thoracic Surgery Database risk adjustment model. J Thorac Cardiovasc Surg 2009;137(3):587–95 [discussion 596].
19. Onaitis MW, Furnary AP, Kosinski AS, et al. Prediction of long-term survival after lung cancer surgery for elderly patients in the society of thoracic surgeons general thoracic surgery database. Ann Thorac Surg 2018;105(1):309–16.
20. Jacobs JP, Edwards FH, Shahian DM, et al. Successful linking of the Society of Thoracic Surgeons adult cardiac surgery database to Centers for Medicare and Medicaid Services Medicare data. Ann Thorac Surg 2010;90(4):1150–6 [discussion 1156–7].
21. Jacobs JP, Edwards FH, Shahian DM, et al. Successful linking of the Society of Thoracic Surgeons database to social security data to examine survival after cardiac operations. Ann Thorac Surg 2011; 92(1):32–7 [discussion 38–9].
22. Savitch SL, Grenda TR, Scott W, et al. Racial disparities in rates of surgery for esophageal cancer: a study from the national cancer database. J Gastrointest Surg 2021;25(3):581–92.
23. Barsky AR, Ahern CA, Venigalla S, et al. Gender-based disparities in receipt of care and survival in malignant pleural mesothelioma. Clin Lung Cancer 2020;21(6):e583–91.

24. Cassidy RJ, Zhang X, Switchenko JM, et al. Health care disparities among octogenarians and nonagenarians with stage III lung cancer. Cancer 2018; 124(4):775–84.

25. Mallin K, Browner A, Palis B, et al. Incident cases captured in the national cancer database compared with those in U.S. population based central cancer registries in 2012-2014. Ann Surg Oncol 2019; 26(6):1604–12.

26. Bleicher RJ, Ruth K, Sigurdson ER, et al. Time to surgery and breast cancer survival in the United States. JAMA Oncol 2016;2(3):330–9.

27. Tong BC, Kim S, Kosinski A, et al. Penetration, completeness, and representativeness of the society of thoracic surgeons general thoracic surgery database for lobectomy. Ann Thorac Surg 2019; 107(3):897–902.

28. Jacobs JP, Shahian DM, He X, et al. Penetration, completeness, and representativeness of the society of thoracic surgeons adult cardiac surgery database. Ann Thorac Surg 2016;101(1):33–41 [discussion 41].

29. Zhou N, Corsini EM, Jin S, et al. Advanced data analytics for clinical research part I: what are the tools? Innovations (Phila) 2020;15(2):114–9.

30. Zhou N, Corsini EM, Jin S, et al. Advanced data analytics for clinical research part II: application to cardiothoracic surgery. Innovations (Phila) 2020; 15(2):155–62.

31. Atay SM, Correa AM, Hofstetter WL, et al. Perioperative outcomes of patients undergoing lobectomy on clopidogrel. Ann Thorac Surg 2017;104(6):1821–8.

32. Van Haren RM, Correa AM, Sepesi B, et al. Ground glass lesions on chest imaging: evaluation of reported incidence in cancer patients using natural language processing. Ann Thorac Surg 2019; 107(3):936–40.

33. Shewale JB, Nelson DB, Rice DC, et al. Natural history of ground-glass lesions among patients with previous lung cancer. Ann Thorac Surg 2018; 105(6):1671–7.

34. Lacson R, Wang A, Cochon L, et al. Factors associated with optimal follow-up in women with BI-RADS 3 breast findings. J Am Coll Radiol 2020;17(4):469–74.

35. OCEBM Levels of Evidence Working Group. The oxford levels of evidence 2. Oxford Centre for Evidence-Based Medicine. Available at: https://www.cebm.ox.ac.uk/resources/levels-of-evidence/ocebm-levels-of-evidence. Accessed March 15, 2021.

36. Jiang T, Bai Y, Zhou F, et al. Clinical value of neutrophil-to-lymphocyte ratio in patients with non-small-cell lung cancer treated with PD-1/PD-L1 inhibitors. Lung Cancer 2019;130:76–83.

37. Ludmir EB, Mainwaring W, Lin TA, et al. Factors associated with age disparities among cancer clinical trial participants. JAMA Oncol 2019;5(12):1769–73.

38. Ludmir EB, Subbiah IM, Mainwaring W, et al. Decreasing incidence of upper age restriction enrollment criteria among cancer clinical trials. J Geriatr Oncol 2020;11(3):451–4.

39. Ludmir EB, Fuller CD, Moningi S, et al. Sex-based disparities among cancer clinical trial participants. J Natl Cancer Inst 2020;112(2):211–3.

40. Grant SR, Lin TA, Miller AB, et al. Racial and ethnic disparities among participants in US-based phase 3 randomized cancer clinical trials. JNCI Cancer Spectr 2020;4(5):pkaa060.

41. Loree JM, Anand S, Dasari A, et al. Disparity of race reporting and representation in clinical trials leading to cancer drug approvals from 2008 to 2018. JAMA Oncol 2019;5(10):e191870.

42. Doroshow DB, Sanmamed MF, Hastings K, et al. Immunotherapy in non-small cell lung cancer: facts and hopes. Clin Cancer Res 2019;25(15):4592–602.

43. Owen D, Chaft JE. Immunotherapy in surgically resectable non-small cell lung cancer. J Thorac Dis 2018;10(Suppl 3):S404–11.

44. Wu YL, Tsuboi M, He J, et al. Osimertinib in resected EGFR-mutated non-small-cell lung cancer. N Engl J Med 2020;383(18):1711–23.

45. Kim J, Bowlby R, Mungall AJ, et al. Integrated genomic characterization of oesophageal carcinoma. Nature 2017;541(7636):169–75.

46. Behrens C, Rocha P, Parra ER, et al. Female gender predicts augmented immune infiltration in lung adenocarcinoma. Clin Lung Cancer 2021;22(3):e415–24.

47. Arauz RF, Byun JS, Tandon M, et al. Whole-exome profiling of NSCLC among African Americans. J Thorac Oncol 2020;15(12):1880–92.

48. Mitchell KA, Nichols N, Tang W, et al. Recurrent PTPRT/JAK2 mutations in lung adenocarcinoma among African Americans. Nat Commun 2019; 10(1):5735.

49. Mitchell KA, Zingone A, Toulabi L, et al. Comparative transcriptome profiling reveals coding and noncoding RNA differences in NSCLC from African Americans and European Americans. Clin Cancer Res 2017;23(23):7412–25.

50. Deveaux AE, Allen TA, Al Abo M, et al. RNA splicing and aggregate gene expression differences in lung squamous cell carcinoma between patients of West African and European ancestry. Lung Cancer 2021; 153:90–8.

51. Lusk CM, Watza D, Dyson G, et al. Profiling the mutational landscape in known driver genes and novel genes in African American non-small cell lung cancer patients. Clin Cancer Res 2019; 25(14):4300–8.

52. Steuer CE, Behera M, Berry L, et al. Role of race in oncogenic driver prevalence and outcomes in lung

adenocarcinoma: results from the Lung Cancer Mutation Consortium. Cancer 2016;122(5):766–72.

53. Campbell JD, Lathan C, Sholl L, et al. Comparison of prevalence and types of mutations in lung cancers among black and white populations. JAMA Oncol 2017;3(6):801–9.

54. Choudhury NJ, Eghtesad M, Kadri S, et al. Fewer actionable mutations but higher tumor mutational burden characterizes NSCLC in black patients at an urban academic medical center. Oncotarget 2019;10(56):5817–23.

55. Vodicka E, Kim K, Devine EB, et al. Inclusion of patient-reported outcome measures in registered clinical trials: evidence from ClinicalTrials.gov (2007–2013). Contemp Clin Trials 2015;43:1–9.

56. Philip EJ, Coups EJ, Feinstein MB, et al. Physical activity preferences of early-stage lung cancer survivors. Support Care Cancer 2014;22(2):495–502.

57. Fayanju OM, Ren Y, Stashko I, et al. Patient-reported causes of distress predict disparities in time to evaluation and time to treatment after breast cancer diagnosis. Cancer 2021;127(5):757–68.

58. Smith AB, Samuel CA, McCabe SD, et al. Feasibility and delivery of patient-reported outcomes in clinical practice among racially diverse bladder and prostate cancer patients. Urol Oncol 2021;39(1):77. e71–8.

59. Grant SR, Noticewala SS, Mainwaring W, et al. Non-English language validation of patient-reported outcome measures in cancer clinical trials. Support Care Cancer 2020;28(6):2503–5.

Social Disparities in Thoracic Surgery Education

Luis A. Godoy, MD[a],*, Elise Hill, MD[b], David T. Cooke, MD[a]

KEYWORDS

• Disparities • Diversity • Inclusion • Workforce • Mentorship • Pipeline

KEY POINTS

- Heart and lung disease are leading factors affecting morbidity and mortality in Black/African Americans and Latinos/Hispanics.
- The US population is the most diverse than it has ever been and will continue to diversify based on Census projections.
- Women and URM lack proportionate membership in the CT surgery trainees, workforce, and leadership.
- There is a lack of mentors and role models within the CT surgery specialty.
- Recruitment efforts should begin earlier than previously thought, most importantly, in the preclinical years.

INTRODUCTION: RACIAL/ETHNIC AND GENDER HEALTH DISPARITIES

In the United States, there is a long history of differences in access to medical care by race and ethnicity.[1] Heart and lung disease are leading factors affecting morbidity and mortality in Black/African Americans and Latinos/Hispanics.[2] Notably, although lung cancer is the number one killer of Black/African Americans, and number 2 killer of Latinos/Hispanics,[3,4] Black/African Americans are less likely to receive surgery for lung cancer than other groups.[5]

Similarly, gender disparities are well documented. Lung cancer and heart disease are the leading causes of death among US women.[6] Despite improvements in surgical and pharmaceutical interventions, women have increased risk for morbidity and mortality after multiple types of cardiac surgery.[7]

Data released by the US Census Bureau in 2018 estimated that about 40% of Americans identified as racial or ethnic minorities (**Fig. 1**).[8,9] Although at the time of this, writing the most recent 2020 Census data is being processed, it is expected to reveal a more diverse nation than was previously projected. Looking at the data for younger generations, especially those under the age of 18, it shows that these younger age groups are composed of approximately 50% minorities (see **Fig. 1**).[8,9] What this implies is that the population will undoubtedly become more diverse as the population ages.

With heart and lung disease being the leading factors affecting morbidity and mortality in these groups, cardiothoracic (CT) surgeons are uniquely positioned to positively affect these health outcomes. As the population becomes more diverse, it is imperative that the composition of the workforce diversify as well. This includes the

---

[a] Division of General Thoracic Surgery, Department of Surgery, University of California, Davis Health, North Addition Office Building, 2335 Stockton Boulevard, Suite 6123, Sacramento, CA 95817-2214, USA;
[b] Department of Surgery, University of California, Davis Health, North Addition Office Building, 2335 Stockton Boulevard, Suite 6123, Sacramento, CA 95817-2214, USA
* Corresponding author.
E-mail address: lagodoy@ucdavis.edu

Thorac Surg Clin 32 (2022) 91–102
https://doi.org/10.1016/j.thorsurg.2021.09.010
1547-4127/22/© 2021 Elsevier Inc. All rights reserved.

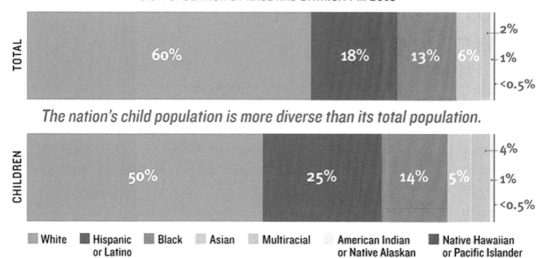

Fig. 1. US population by race and ethnicity in 2018. (*From* The Annie E. Casey Foundation. What the Data Say About Race, Ethnicity and American Youth. Year. Available at: https://www.aecf.org/blog/what-the-data-say-about-race-ethnicity-and-american-youth Accessed April 20, 2021.)

diversification of the educational pipeline into CT surgery. This article will discuss the current state of the pipeline, barriers faced, and suggestions for improvement.

COMPOSITION OF THE CT SURGERY FACULTY/TRAINEE WORKFORCE

Despite an ever-diversifying US population, women, and underrepresented minorities (URM) lack proportionate membership in the CT surgery workforce. A survey conducted by the American College of Surgeons (ACS) in 2009 identified CT surgery as the surgical specialty practiced by the oldest surgeons as a group with 53.9% of practicing CT surgeons older than 55 year old.[10] This was corroborated by the 2014 Society of Thoracic Surgeons (STS) Workforce Report which revealed that the median age of the active US CT surgeon was 54 years. In addition, it also demonstrated that women comprised only 6.3% of adult cardiac, 6.1% of congenital heart, and 11.8% of general thoracic surgeons.[11] Racial and ethnic demographic data were not presented. These striking results highlight a deficit within our specialty and foreshadows a shrinking of the CT surgery workforce that will be compounded by a lack of diversity as the workforce ages.

To analyze the composition of the current workforce, Erkmen and colleagues queried the Accreditation Council for Graduate Medical Education (ACGME) and Association of American Medical Colleges (AAMC) databases for racial/ethnic and gender demographics of residents and

faculty. Women and racial/ethnic minorities were found to be underrepresented among trainees and faculty in academic CT surgery than general surgery and medicine overall (**Fig. 2**).[12] Black/African American and Latino/Hispanic physicians composed only 4% and 5% of the CT surgery residents, respectively.[12]

DISPARITIES IN THE PIPELINE

A contributing factor to the lack of diversity within CT surgery may be because the numbers of URM medical school applicants and graduates continue to be low. According to the AAMC, the percentages of medical school graduates by race and ethnicity have also remained consistent over time with only 4.6% Black/African American and 5.7% Latino/Hispanic medical school graduates in 2016.[13] As the number of URM medical school graduates remain consistently low, diverse applicants to CT surgery will also continue to remain low.

The problem is not solely within the pipeline. In 2019, according to the data released by the AAMC women now comprised most of the enrolled US medical students.[14] The proportion of women students has been rising over recent years, from 46.9% in 2015%, 49.5% in 2018%, and 50.5% in 2019.[14] This progressive trend, however, has not carried over into CT surgery training programs and vis-à-vis the CT surgery workforce.

Another problem with recruitment is the overall lack of exposure to CT surgery. Few URM medical school matriculants decide to pursue surgical

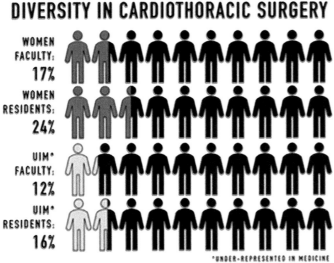

Fig. 2. Proportion of women and racial/ethnic minorities among trainees and faculty in academic CT surgery. (*From* Ortmeyer KA, Raman V, Tiko-Okoye C, Espinosa J, Cooke DT, Erkmen CP. Women and Minorities Underrepresented in Academic Cardiothoracic Surgery: It's Time for Next Steps. Ann Thorac Surg. 2020 Nov 5:S0003–4975(20)31851–8.)

careers. Of those that do decide to choose general surgery, very few have significant exposure to CT surgery. The current ACGME general surgery case requirements have minimal thoracic surgical cases required and zero cardiac surgery requirements (**Fig. 3**).[15] As work hour restrictions have been implemented, programs have streamlined resident rotations to meet required cases. As such, CT surgery rotations are no longer required. With such limited exposure to CTS, it is no surprise that trainees shy away from CT surgery as a career option. Potential URM and

Category			Minimum
Skin, Soft Tissue			25
Breast			40
	Mastectomy		5
	Axilla		5
Head and Neck			25
Alimentary Tract			180
	Esophagus		5
	Stomach		15
	Small Intestine		25
	Large Intestine		40
	Appendix		40
	Anorectal		20
Thoracic Surgery			20
	Thoracotomy		5
Cardiac Surgery			0

Fig. 3. Acgme defined category minimum numbers for general surgery residents. (*From* Accreditation Council for Graduate Medical Education (ACGME). Defined Category Minimum Numbers for General Surgery Residents and Credit Role Review Committee for Surgery. Available at: https://www.acgme.org/Portals/0/DefinedCategoryMinimumNumbersforGeneralSurgeryResidentsandCreditRole.pdf.)

women candidates may interpret the current absence of diversity in CT surgery as exclusive and unwelcoming and may choose to apply to more inclusive fields. In addition, the lack of women and URM faculty members may translate into a lack of mentorship and sponsorship of potential candidates.

In addition to problems with filling the pipeline and recruitment, there is also a problem with retention. Davis and Yang looked at the National Resident Matching Program (NRMP) data and identified 147 individuals that applied to CT surgery Integrated Programs (IP) from 2008 to 2011 and were unmatched in CT surgery IP but matched into general surgery. Only 20 of those individuals (14%) ended up in CT surgery fellowship programs (**Fig. 4**).[16] This was a surprising finding given that IP applicants typically have demonstrated a strong interest in CT surgery at the time of their application. As mentioned earlier, it is thought part of the problem is the limited exposure to CT surgery as general surgery trainees.

POSSIBLE SOLUTIONS

In 2014, STS Workforce Report, Ikonomidis and colleagues reported that 48% of survey respondents identified their decision to pursue a career in CT surgery was made before or in medical school.[11] Similarly, Meza and colleagues conducted a survey of IP surgery program applicants. In their survey, a specific question was asked; *When did you develop an interest in CT Surgery?* Interestingly, 61% of respondents

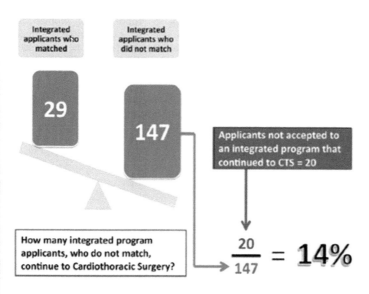

Fig. 4. Unmatched Integrated program applicants who continued to cardiothoracic surgery, 2008 to 2011. *(From* Davis TA, Yang SC. Unmatched Integrated Cardiothoracic Surgery Program Applicants: Where Do They End Up? Ann Thorac Surg. 2018 Nov;106(5):1556–1560.)

stated that they had an interest in CT surgery before clinical clerkships and 93% tailored their clinical education to meet that interest (**Fig. 5**).[17] These survey results suggest that recruitment must start earlier than residency. Efforts to fill the pipeline must start earlier than previously thought. We should target pipeline efforts to the preclinical years as this is when most applicants decide on a specialty. We should focus our active recruitment strategies toward underrepresented in medicine-specific organizations and clubs such as Latino Medical Student Association (LMSA), Student National Medical Association (SNMA), Women in Medicine (WIM), and so forth. In addition, it has been shown that early mentorship is crucial to fostering an interest in CT surgery. This must start early in the premedical years, possibly even as early as high school.

In addition, the retention of interested applicants is just as important. After application cycles, it is important to continue to engage IP applicants to keep them interested in CT surgery. This can be

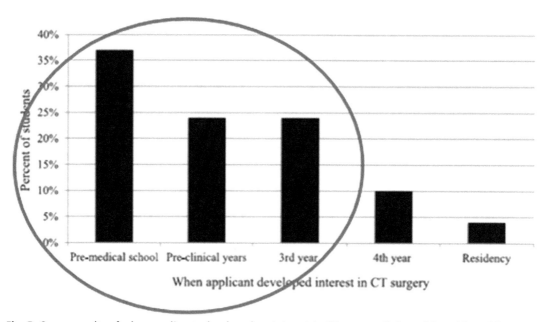

Fig. 5. Survey results of when applicants developed an interest in CT surgery. *(Adapted from* Meza JM, Rectenwald JE, Reddy RM. The bias against integrated thoracic surgery residency applicants during general surgery interviews. Ann Thorac Surg. 2015 Apr;99(4):1206–12.)

conducted by providing research opportunities for those residents who fail to match into IP training programs and match into general surgery. We can also offer CT surgery electives for general surgery residents who are interested in the specialty.

The STS Workforce on Diversity and Inclusion was created to address the needs of our specialty to better reflect and understand (cultural competence) our evolving communities. These values are held by many STS members who view achieving a diverse CT surgery workforce as important.[18] It is crucial that we as a specialty create mechanisms to keep these talented diverse individuals within the pipeline. To do so, we must create an environment that is welcoming and create a culture of inclusion within our institutions.

CREATING A CULTURE OF INCLUSION

As previously discussed, there is a lack of representation among women and URM in the CT surgery workforce. We have delineated steps that can recruit a more diverse workforce. Attention must now be turned to the strategies and tools that can be used to create an atmosphere of inclusion, which is critical to the retention of diverse staff and trainees. Pursuant to this goal, the STS created a Task Force, later developed into a Workforce on Diversity and Inclusion which was tasked with creating an environment of diversity and inclusion both within the STS and the CT surgery specialty overall. The mission and goals of the STS Task Force are shown in **Table 1**.[18]

To begin to address issues of diversity and inclusion within any institution, the subject must first be defined. According to Merriam-Webster, diversity is defined as "the condition of having or being composed of different elements especially: the inclusion of different types of people (such as people of different races or cultures) in a group or organization."[19] The definition of inclusion is "the act or practice of including and accommodating people who have historically been excluded (as because of their race, gender, sexuality or ability)."[20]

Once a particular entity has defined what diversity and inclusion means within the context of their institution, a baseline assessment of thoughts and perceptions surrounding the matter must be defined.

The STS Task Force conducted a climate survey from November 2017 to January 2018. The survey was emailed to 5158 STS members, with a 9.3% response rate. The responders were asked to self-identify their professional roles, including the option of "CT surgery workforce decision makers", that is, program directors, department chair, and so forth. Although the low response rate precludes the scientific generalizability of the results, conclusions can be drawn on the attitudes and perceptions many of the members of STS hold regarding issues of diversity and inclusion. **Table 2** summarizes the results of the survey.[18]

Notably across the board, both "all respondents" and those identified as "decision makers" viewed the importance of achieving URM and gender diversity as important to extremely important. More interestingly are the responses to the question "What are some barriers to diversity and/or inclusion within CT Surgery?" As seen in **Table 3**, while the number one response from the responders that identified as decision makers, white/Caucasian and male was "Lifestyle concerns of a career in CT surgery as they pertain to family planning", this did not hold true for women and minorities.[18] Among women and minorities, the top reasons were either a lack of CT surgery exposure to URM and/or women medical students and surgical residents or few URM and/or women

Table 1	Mission, vision, and goals of the society of thoracic surgeons task force on diversity and inclusion	
Mission	The STS Task Force on Diversity and Inclusion will cultivate an environment of inclusion and diversity within the STS as well as the cardiothoracic surgical specialty.
Vision	A workforce equipped to care for diverse populations nationally and internationally.
Goals	• Establish an STS Task Force to advise the STS and develop diversity and inclusion-related initiatives and activities.
	• Partner with leaders within centers of excellence, academic units, and societies to provide educational offerings to improve cultural competence, health disparities, and health equity within cardiothoracic clinical, scientific, education, and advocacy environments.
	• Foster a climate that possesses respect, integrity, inclusion, and open dialogue between members.

STS, The Society of Thoracic Surgeons.
From Cooke DT, Olive J, Godoy L, Preventza O, Mathisen DJ, Prager RL. The Importance of a Diverse Specialty: Introducing the STS Workforce on Diversity and Inclusion. Ann Thorac Surg. 2019 Oct;108(4):1000 - 1005.

Table 2
The society of thoracic surgeon members views on the importance of underrepresented minority and gender diversity

Question	Extremely Important/ Important % (n)	Not at All Important/Not Important %<n)	Neither Important nor Not Important % (n)	1 Don't Know %(n)
How important Is it (all respondents):				
For the cardiothoracic surgery, workforce to achieve a representative group of minorities?	67.0 (320)	15.1 (72)	16.7 (80)	13(6)
To achieve a representative group of women in the cardiothoracic surgery workforce?	68.8 (329)	13.8 (66)	16.7 (80)	0.6 (3)
To have a representative group of minority trainees entering cardiothoracic surgery?	67.2 (322)	14.0 (67)	17.5 (84)	13 (6)
To have a representative group of women trainees entering cardiothoracic surgery?	68.4 (326)	14.7 (70)	15.9 (76)	1.1 (5)
How important is it (cardiothoracic surgery workforce decision makers):				
For the cardiothoracic surgery workforce to achieve a representative group of minorities?	64.9 (61)	18.1 (17)	10.1 (9)	1.1 (1)
To achieve a representative group of women in the cardiothoracic surgery workforce?	65.6 (61)	183 (17)	16.1 (15)	0.0 (0)
To have a representative group of minority trainees entering cardiothoracic surgery?	66.0 (62)	18.1 (17)	14.9 (14)	1.1 (1)
To have a representative group of women trainees entering cardiothoracic surgery?	67.0 (63)	19.2 (18)	12.8(12)	1.1 (1)

From Cooke DT, Olive J, Godoy L, Preventza O, Mathisen DJ, Prager RL. The Importance of a Diverse Specialty: Introducing the STS Workforce on Diversity and Inclusion. Ann Thorac Surg. 2019 Oct;108(4):1000 - 1005.

CT surgery mentors and role models. This data provides salient insight into perception versus reality and can act as a guide to creating a truly inclusive environment that fosters both the recruitment and retention of a diverse CT surgery workforce.[19]

BIAS AS A THREAT TO INCLUSIVITY

One of the major barriers to the creation of an inclusive environment is the presence of implicit and explicit bias within the CT specialty and health care overall. Exposure to this negative bias lowers confidence, strains camaraderie, and prevents those individuals from thriving in their chosen field. It is antithetical to inclusion and must be eradicated. The STS Workforce on Diversity and Inclusion published a report on the literature regarding gender and race-related bias experienced by surgical trainees and members of the CT surgery workforce.[21] They provided results from a survey that was completed on the topic to get a baseline for whereby the specialty is currently on this issue, to better provide a path forward. Implicit bias testing shows that, among patients and medical

Table 3
Top 3 responses to the Question: "What are some of the barriers to diversity and/or inclusion within cardiothoracic surgery?"

All Respondents (n = 330)	CT Surgery Workforce Decision Makers (n = 74)	Black/African/African American (n = 23)	Latino/Hispanic (n = 29)
1. Few underrepresented minority and/or women CT surgery mentors and role models 2. Lifestyle concern of a career in CT surgery as they pertain to family planning 3. A lack of CT surgery exposure to underrepresented minority and/or women medical students and surgical residents	1. Lifestyle concerns of a career in CT surgery as they pertain to family planning 2. Few underrepresented minority and/or women CT surgery mentors and role models 3. A lack of CT surgery exposure to underrepresented minority and/or women medical students and surgical residents	1. Few underrepresented minority and/or women CT surgery mentors and role models 2. A lack of CT surgery exposure to underrepresented minority and/or women medical students and surgical residents 3. Perceptions of unconscious bias by CT surgery residency programs toward underrepresented minority and/or women applicants	1. A lack of CT surgery exposure to underrepresented minority and/or women medical students and surgical residents 2. Few underrepresented minority and/or women CT surgery mentors and role models 3. Perceptions of unconscious bias by CT surgery residency programs toward underrepresented minority and/or women applicants

Asian/Last Asian/South Asian (n = 71)	White/Caucasian (n = 228)	Female (n = 66)	Male (n = 230)
1. Few underrepresented minority and/or women CT surgery mentors and role models 2. Perceptions of unconscious bias by CT surgery leadership toward potential underrepresented minority and/or women faculty and staff 3. Lifestyle concerns of a carver in CT surgery as they pertain to family planning	1. Lifestyle concerns of a career in CT surgery as they pertain to family planning 2. Few underrepresented minority and/or women CT surgery mentors and role models 3. A lack of CT surgery exposure to underrepresented minority and/or women medical students and surgical residents	1. Few underrepresented minority and/or women CT surgery mentors and role models 2. Perceptions of unconscious bias by CT surgery leadership toward potential underrepresented minority and/or women faculty and staff 3. A lack of CT surgery exposure to underrepresented minority and/or women medical students and surgical residents	1. Lifestyle concerns of a career in CT surgery as they pertain to family planning 2. Few underrepresented minority and/or women CT surgery mentors and role models 3. A lack of CT surgery exposure to underrepresented minority and/or women medical students and surgical residents

Abbreviations: CT, cardiothoracic STS, The Society of Thoracic Surgeons
From Cooke DT, Olive J, Godoy L, Preventza O, Mathisen DJ, Prager RL. The Importance of a Diverse Specialty: Introducing the STS Workforce on Diversity and Inclusion. Ann Thorac Surg. 2019 Oct;108(4):1000 - 1005.

professionals, there is a stronger association of the male gender with both career and surgery.[22] In addition, a study aimed at the evaluation of the effect of implicit bias on leadership positions found that all faculty held a slight preference for men versus women in leadership positions, and this preference was strongest in the older, male faculty.[23] In looking at female leadership within the STS, only 1 woman has ever held the position of president (posthumously) and a mere 2 of 19 members of the board of directors are women. This lack of representation at the leadership diminishes cognitive perspective and may reinforce implicit biases. In practice, this is demonstrated by tangible negative effects felt by female surgical trainees, including less operating autonomy by both resident and attending surgeons.[24] The prevalence of racial bias and its effect on training and entry into the surgical workforce is well documented. Significant bias, white over black, was demonstrated during an implicit bias test administered to the admissions committee of a prominent medical school.[25] A direct link between implicit bias and dissatisfaction of diverse residents is identified by Wong and colleagues[26] whereby 4339 surgical residents were surveyed during the American Board of Surgery In-Training Examination. The results show that minority residents report fewer positive relationships with peers and faculty, and that Black and Asian residents reported more frequently that they believed their attendings would think less of them if they asked for help. This data displays the very real threat that bias poses to creating an inclusive environment. Based on a small study by Liebschutz and colleagues[27] that detailed the discriminatory experience of 19 black residents, a research team, led by Osseo-Assare, conducted qualitative interviews with more than two dozen URM medical and surgical residents. Three main conclusions were drawn from the interviews. First, microaggressions were experienced daily, defined as "subtle snubs, slights, and insults directed toward minorities, as well as to women and other historically stigmatized groups, that implicitly communicate or at least engender hostility." Second, URM residents relayed being asked and/or expected to serve as ambassadors to assist with issues of diversity in their institutions. Third, the residents reported a prevailing sense of dissociation between their professional and personal identities. These residents also described commonly being mistaken for nonmedical staff, an experience that serves to undermine confidence and feeling of belonging.[28]

To bring the focus specifically to the STS and members' experiences with implicit bias, the Task Force queried 5158 members with 481 responses. The question asked to assess implicit and explicit bias was "Have you ever felt unfairly treated by your colleagues within the larger CT professional community because of your race/ethnicity/gender/sexual orientation/religion/age/disability status?" Key findings from this survey are that most of the female (69.7%) and Black (82.6%) respondents answered yes than few yes respondents by other demographic groups (**Table 4**).[21] As stated before, the effect of bias on degrading culture of inclusion cannot be overstated. To move the CT surgery specialty toward an inclusive institution, implicit and explicit bias must be eradicated.

START WITH A CHECKLIST

A recent article by Ortmeyer *and colleagues* aimed to provide a checklist for the development of program-specific diversity and inclusion policy within CT surgery programs.[29] Recommendations were developed from a comprehensive review of hundreds of articles in diversity and inclusion within the surgical sector, as well as some guidance from other industries such as psychology, sociology, and the private sector. Contributions were considered from the ACGME, AAMC, the ACS, the American Surgical Association (ASA), and various other sources. Following the review of these publications, 5 themes emerged, as shown in **Fig. 6** and summarized with the acronym G.O.A.L.S. (goals, organizational change, advocacy, diversity literacy, and sustainability).[29]

As with any quality improvement project, the first step is establishing specific goals. Begin with the creation of a mission statement that defines the organizations' commitment to diversity and inclusion. Discuss whereby the organization would like to be in a set amount of time and formalize this with a vision statement. Define how the program intends to measure successes and failures related to its goals. For example, collect the numbers of URM and woman applicants, interviewees, and subsequent trainees. Recall that the number one barrier to diversity in CT surgery for URM and women, based on the STS Task Force climate survey, was the lack of exposure to CT surgery and lack of role models/mentors. Acknowledge the importance of addressing this by setting goals for faculty recruitment and retention as well. Create an environment of inclusion by examining compensation systems, promotion, and evaluation for evidence of bias. Once discrete goals have been established, including methods to evaluate successes and failures, share this commitment with current program members, and

Table 4
The Society of thoracic surgeons' workforce on diversity and inclusion climate survey

| Respondents | Have you ever felt unfairly treated (eg, marginalized, mistreated, harassed excluded, bullied, not promoted, diminished) by your colleagues within the Larger cardiothoracic professional community because of your race/ethnicity/gender/sexual orientation/religion/age/disability status? | | |
	Yes % (n)	*No.* % (n)	I Don't Know, % (n)
All respondents	33.8(161)	62.1 (296)	4.2 (20)
Female	69.7 (53)	23.7(18)	6.6 (5)
Male	24.7 (75)	72.0 (219)	3.3 (10)
Black/African/African American	82.6(19)	17.4 (4)	0.0 (0)
White/Caucasian	269 (61)	71.8 (163)	13(3)
Latino/Hispanic	24.1 (7)	72.4(21)	35(1)
Asian/East Asian/South Asian	39.4 (28)	47.9 (34)	12.7 (9)
CT surgery workforce decision makers	28.7 (27)	70.2 (66)	1.1 (1)

From Erhunmwunsee L, Backhus LM, Godoy L, Edwards MA, Cooke DT. Report from the Workforce on Diversity and Inclusion-The Society of Thoracic Surgeons Members' Bias Experiences. Ann Thorac Surg. 2019 Nov;108(5):1287 - 1291.

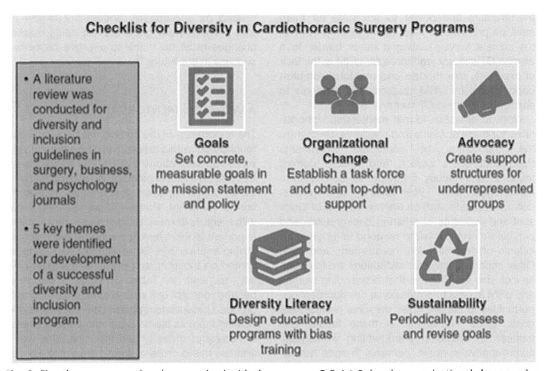

Fig. 6. Five themes emerged and summarized with the acronym G.O.A.L.S. (goals, organizational change, advocacy, diversity literacy, and sustainability). *(From* Ortmeyer KA, Raman V, Tiko-Okoye CS, Espinosa JA, Cooke DT, Starnes SL, Erkmen CP. Goals, organizational change, advocacy, diversity literacy, and sustainability: A checklist for diversity in cardiothoracic surgery training programs. J Thorac Cardiovasc Surg. 2020 Dec 3:S0022-5223(20) 33199-8.)

provide the information to prospective trainees and staff. Demonstrate commitment to set goals by dedicating resources aimed at the production of scholarly work pertaining to diversity and inclusion initiatives within the program; share successes and failures in peer-reviewed publications and at national meetings to assist in the eradication of structural bias within CT surgery.

Institutional change requires organizational change and buy-in from institutional leadership. Garner this support by establishing a specific Task Force aimed at achieving the mission of the institution. Empower the Task Force by providing recognition and consider compensation for members. This Task Force should analyze barriers to diversity and inclusion within their institution, develop actionable goals, and identify additional investments needed to obtain such goals. Connect the Task Force with existing diversity and inclusion groups within other departments for synergistic progress. Use available resources from other offices to advance a culture of diversity and inclusion within CT surgery. For example, many Diversity and Inclusion Offices provide funding for URM subinternships, inclusion training, and support for URM faculty and trainees. To foster an inclusive environment for URM and women faculty, trainees, and recruits, a support system with the structure and power to advocate for them must be prioritized. Once again, bearing in mind the climate survey stating a major barrier to a diverse CT surgery workforce for URM is the lack of exposure, role models and mentors, establish opportunities for URM students and residents to shadow or intern in CT surgery.

Work to establish formal mentorship opportunities for these students and residents. Recognize the importance of continued mentorship throughout one's career, and ensure current trainees, and faculty continue to benefit from mentorship, both inter-cultural and cross-cultural. Educate staff on the mentorship of junior staff and residents of differing backgrounds and provide training on how to respond to reported incidents of discrimination, harassment, and bias. Other important ways for institutions are to create an inclusive environment that is providing women and URM access to professional development opportunities to achieve their personal professional goals. Show investment in these faculty and trainees by providing grant writing workshops, administrative support, personal finance education, and clear and transparent paths for advancement. Although working toward a more diverse workforce, a program can create inclusion through the acknowledgment of the weighty loneliness URM faculty and trainees may feel, especially due to national structural racism, such as unfair and life-threatening policing and the disproportional effects of COVID-19 on communities of color. The feelings of diverse colleagues must be recognized by institutional leadership and support groups and/or safe spaces should be provided. Should this not be possible due to the current demographic make-up of the program, dedicated cross-program, or technological conferencing should be considered to fill this gap. The development of educational programs aimed at improving the diversity and inclusion literacy of a department is paramount to mitigating the structural bias that destroys inclusivity. Historical perspective and empirical data should be provided to the entire department to emphasize the prevalence of discrimination and bias and show the importance of diversity in an organization's success. All employees should be educated on the definitions of discrimination, microaggression, and implicit bias. Implicit bias training should be formally implemented, to include the evaluation of individual implicit bias evaluation with tools like the Harvard Implicit Association Test.[30]

Finally, sustainability must be acknowledged as an important part of the implementation of any diversity and inclusion program. Goals should be systematically evaluated at least annually and revised as appropriate. Should the review find that previously set goals are not being reached, changes must be made to improve chances of success in the future.[29]

A WORD ON MENTORSHIP

The importance of mentorship has been previously touched on in this article. Based on the data presented on perceptions, by URM and female trainees that there is a lack of mentors and role models within the CT surgery specialty, it is clear that representation is important. Partnering trainees and faculty with mentors from within their demographic can be important to them feeling a sense of belonging and having a safe space. Other data that have been presented on thoughts and opinions regarding diversity, as seen in **Table 3**, show a disconnect between perceptions among different demographic groups. Understanding these differences and overcoming them as teams is paramount to success in the arena of diversity and inclusion. One way to address this is cross-cultural mentorship. By cultivating relationships between people with different backgrounds, both parties will benefit by better understanding whereby the other is coming from. This may lead to decreased misconceptions about the reasons causing failure in diversity and/or inclusion, allowing interventions to be targeted on the appropriate issues.

SUMMARY

Despite an ever-diversifying US population, women, and URM lack proportionate membership in the CT surgery workforce and leadership. As members of the specialty, we are in an influential position that can help shape the future demographics of our specialty. Although the applicant pool is small, we as members of this specialty are in a unique position to help mentor and guide these potential applicants. We can do so by creating a welcoming culture, by providing mentorship and exposure, all of which have been shown to be critical aspects in specialty choice. It is imperative that we as a specialty create mechanisms to keep these talented individuals within the pipeline and within the workforce. If CT surgery is to continue to advance forward and attract the brightest, most skilled, and innovative people, we as members of this group must invite, encourage, and guide qualified individuals from all races, cultures, genders, sexual orientation, and experiences to join us.

CLINICS CARE POINTS

- Participate in medical school and residency admissions committees and advocate for diversity and inclusion
- Reach out to medical student groups with mentorship opportunities during preclinical years
- Offer research opportunities and mentor general surgery residents at your institution
- Use the 5 key components for the development of successful diversity and inclusion program

DISCLOSURE

The authors have nothing to disclose.

REFERENCES

1. U.S. Department of Health and Human Services (U.S. DHHS). Report of the secretary's task force on black & minority health, vol I. Washington, DC: Executive Summary; 1985.
2. Mozaffarian D, Benjamin EJ, Go AS, et al. Heart disease and stroke statistics—2015 update: a report from the American Heart Association. Circulation 2015;131:e29–322.
3. American Cancer Society. Cancer facts & figures for hispanics/latinos 2018-2020. Atlanta: American Cancer Society, Inc.; 2018.
4. American Cancer Society. Cancer facts & figures for African Americans 2019-2021. Atlanta: American Cancer Society, Inc; 2019.
5. American lung association state of lung cancer 2020. Available at: https://www.lung.org/research/state-of-lung-cancer/racial-and-ethnic-disparities. Accessed December 21, 2020.
6. Centers for Disease Control. Leading causes of death - females - all races and origins - United States. 2017. Available at: https://www.cdc.gov/women/lcod/2017/all-races-origins/index.htm. Accessed April 20, 2021.
7. Bechtel AJ, Huffmyer JL. Gender differences in postoperative outcomes after cardiac surgery. Anesthesiol Clin 2020;38(2):403–15.
8. United States Census Bureau. A more diverse nation; distribution of race and hispanic origin by age groups. Available at: https://www.census.gov/library/visualizations/2019/comm/age-race-distribution.html. Accessed April 20, 2021.
9. The Annie E. Casey Foundation. What the data Say about race, ethnicity and American Youth. Year. Available at: https://www.aecf.org/blog/what-the-data-say-about-race-ethnicity-and-american-youth. Accessed April 20, 2021.
10. ACS Health Policy Research Institute. Surgical workforce in the United States: profile and recent trends. NC: American College of Surgeons Health Policy Research Institute, Chapel Hill; 2010.
11. Ikonomidis JS. The society of thoracic surgeons thoracic surgery practice and access task force: 2014 workforce report. Ann Thorac Surg 2016;102(6):2118–25.
12. Ortmeyer KA, Raman V, Tiko-Okoye C, et al. Women and minorities underrepresented in academic cardiothoracic surgery: it's time for next steps. Ann Thorac Surg 2021;112(4):1349–55.
13. Association of American Medical Colleges. Current trends in medical education. Available at: https://www.aamcdiversityfactsandfigures2016.org/report-section/section-3/. Accessed April 15, 2021.
14. Association of American Medical Colleges. Fall applicant, matriculant, and enrollment data tables. 2019. Available at: https://www.aamc.org/media/38821/download. Accessed April 22, 2021.
15. Accreditation Council for Graduate Medical Education. Defined category minimum numbers for general surgery residents and Credit role review committee for surgery. Available at: https://www.acgme.org/Portals/0/DefinedCategoryMinimumNumbersforGeneralSurgeryResidentsandCreditRole.pdf. Accessed April 21, 2021.

16. Davis TA, Yang SC. Unmatched integrated cardio-thoracic surgery program applicants: where do they end up? Ann Thorac Surg 2018;106(5): 1556–60.

17. Meza JM, Rectenwald JE, Reddy RM. The bias against integrated thoracic surgery residency applicants during general surgery interviews. Ann Thorac Surg 2015;99(4):1206–12.

18. Cooke DT, Olive J, Godoy L, et al. The importance of a diverse specialty: introducing the STS workforce on diversity and inclusion. Ann Thorac Surg 2019 Oct;108(4):1000–5.

19. Diversity. 2020. In Merriam-webster Dictionary. Available at: https://www.merriam-webster.com/dictionary/diversity. Accessed Octrober 11, 2021.

20. Inclusion. 2020. In Merriam-webster dictionary. Available at: https://www.merriam-webster.com/dictionary/diversity. Accessed Octrober 11, 2021.

21. Erhunmwunsee L, Backhus LM, Godoy LA, et al. "Report from the workforce on diversity and inclusion—the society of thoracic surgeons members' bias experiences. Ann Thorac Surg 2019;108(5): 1287–91.

22. Salles A, Awad M, Goldin L, et al. Estimating implicit and explicit gender bias among health care professionals and surgeons. JAMA Netw Open 2019;2: e196545.

23. Girod S, Fassiotto M, Grewal D, et al. Reducing implicit gender leadership bias in academic medicine with an educational intervention. Acad Med 2016;91: 1143–50.

24. Meyerson SL, Sternbach JM, Zwischenberger JB, et al. The effect of gender on resident autonomy in the operating room. J Surg Educ 2017;74:e111–8.

25. Capers QT, Clinchot D, McDougle L, et al. Implicit racial bias in medical school admissions. Acad Med 2017;92:365–9.

26. Wong RL, Sullivan MC, Yeo HL, et al. Race and surgical residency: results from a national survey of 4339 US general surgery residents. Ann Surg 2013;257:782–7.

27. Liebschutz JM, Darko GO, Finley EP, et al. In the minority: black physicians in residency and their experiences. J Natl Med Assoc 2006;98:1441–8.

28. Osseo-Asare A, Balasuriya L, Huot SJ, et al. Minority resident physicians' views on the role of race/ethnicity in their training experiences in the workplace. JAMA Netw Open 2018;1:e182723.

29. Ortmeyer KA, Raman V, Tiko-Okoye C, et al. Goals, organizational change, advocacy, diversity literacy, and sustainability: a checklist for diversity in cardiothoracic surgery training programs. J Thorac Cardiovasc Surg 2020. https://doi.org/10.1016/j.jtcvs.2020.11.112.

30. Harvard University. Available at: www.projectimplicit.net/. Accessed April 15, 2020.

Social Disparities in the Thoracic Surgery Workforce

DuyKhanh P. Ceppa, MD

KEYWORDS

- Workforce • Disparity • Diversity • Inclusion

KEY POINTS

- Diversity fosters innovation, advances the work environment, and enriches patient care.
- Only 17%, 5%, and 3% of CT surgeons in academia were women, Hispanic, and Black, respectively. (In comparison, the US population is 51%, 18%, and 13% women, Hispanic, and Black, respectively.)
- 70% of women (compared to 25% men), 83% of Black, and 39% of Asian CT surgeons (compared to 27% White/Caucasian CT surgeons) felt they had been unfairly treated based on their gender or race.
- Diversity, equity, and inclusion goals and deliberate initiatives are necessary to eradicate disparities in the CT workforce. Leading organizational changes from the top down is paramount for the sustainability of DEI initiatives.
- Proponents of diversity insist on changes and improvements being based on merit and accomplishments.

INTRODUCTION

The argument for diversity in health care is clear. Diversity fosters innovation, improves the quality of patient care, and decreases health care disparities.[1,2] The surgical workforce, however, lacks in diversity and, more specifically, cardiothoracic (CT) surgery is one of the least diverse medical subspecialties.[3] Recognition of the importance of fostering an inclusive environment has been announced among CT surgery leadership and several diversity, equity, and inclusion (DEI) initiatives are ongoing in our field.[4,5] However, CT surgery remains behind in these issues and obstacles remain before true equity can be achieved.

HISTORY
Women in CT

In 1961, the American Board of Thoracic Surgery (ABTS) certified 3 women in CT surgery.[6] Nina Starr Braunwald (1928–1992) was born in Brooklyn, New York and obtained bachelor and medical degrees from New York University. She was the first woman to train in general surgery at Bellevue and her career led to success at the National Institutes of Health, the University of California San Diego, and Harvard University. Despite her accomplishments (the first successful prosthetic mitral valve replacement in 1960, the development of the Braunwald-Cutter valve and stented aortic homografts, 150 peer-reviewed publications, the

Division of Cardiothoracic Surgery, Indiana University School of Medicine, 545 Barnhill Drive, EH215, Indianapolis, IN 46202, USA
E-mail address: dpceppa@iupui.edu
Twitter: @girlceppa (D.P.C.)

Thorac Surg Clin 32 (2022) 103–109
https://doi.org/10.1016/j.thorsurg.2021.09.002
1547-4127/22/© 2021 Elsevier Inc. All rights reserved.

first female member of the AATS), however, Dr Braunwald spent 24 years as an associate professor and was never promoted to full professor. Ann McKiel, the first woman to complete a thoracic surgery residency, and Nermin Tutunju joined Dr Braunwald in the first class of ABTS-certified women.

The influx of women in CT surgery, thereafter, remained minimal as the number of ABTS-certified women only reach 10 almost 20 years later. In 1984, Dr Leslie Kohman started to invite all women CT surgeons to an informal breakfast during Society of Thoracic Surgeons (STS) and American Association for Thoracic Surgeons (AATS) meetings. These breakfasts provided an environment whereupon attendees could share news, socialize, and network with a focus to mentor young women within the specialty.[7] The Women in Cardiothoracic Surgery (now Women in Thoracic Surgery [WTS]) was officially formed in 1986 with Dr Kohman serving as the first president. The number of women entering our discipline remained low, with the total number of ABTS diplomats reaching only 56 by 1990. In the 1990s and early 2000s, the number of women certifying in thoracic surgery remained below 10 per year, with the average increasing to above 10 per year only after 2005. To date, women in CT surgery average 16 diplomats per year, with 2018 peaking at 27 women passing the certifying examination that year.[6,8]

Three articles on the experiences and status of women in CT surgery have been published, approximately 10 years apart.[8–10] In 1996, Dresler and colleagues[9] noted that while women and men had similar training backgrounds, women were less likely to be full professors (13.6% vs 27%), earned a lower income, and perceived discrimination as hindering their careers more than men. Doningon and colleagues presented an update on women in CT surgery at the 48th annual meeting of the STS. It was reported that more than 50% of women in CT surgery had entered the profession within the prior 10 years, suggesting optimism for continued recruitment of women. In addition, 18% of respondents reported being a full professor, suggesting professional advancement.[10] Most recently, Ceppa and colleagues reported that while the number of women entering the discipline continued to increase at the same rate as in the 2012 update, the percentage of women who were full professors remained similar and women continue to earn lower salaries than men even after accounting for age, years in practice, subspecialty, practice location, and setting.[8] Although it has been 60 years since the first women were certified in CT surgery in the United

States and the number of ABTS-certified women is more than 350, women have yet to achieve equity or equality within the discipline of CT surgery.

Underrepresented Minorities in CT

Unfortunately, the history of underrepresented minority (URM) surgeons is not as well documented. Dr Daniel Hale Williams was a general surgeon who founded the first interracial hospital in the United States. In 1893, he repaired a pericardial wound, constituting the first successful open-heart surgery performed by a Black surgeon.[11] It goes without saying that the legacy of Vivien Thomas (1910–1985) cannot be forgotten. As Dr Alfred Blalock's right hand and laboratory supervisor, despite no formal education, he developed the first surgical treatment for Tetralogy of Fallot and is recognized as having trained generations of cardiac surgeons.[12] His contributions to cardiac surgery are now widely accepted and in honor of his accomplishments, the STS has dedicated an entire symposium on diversity and inclusion during each annual meeting to him. Dr Myra Adele Logan (1908–1977) graduated from medical school in 1933. She completed a residency in surgery at the Harlem Hospital and while she did not formally undergo training in CT surgery, she was the first woman to perform open-heart surgery in 1943 and forged a career in congenital heart surgery.[11] Dr Rosalyn P Scott is the first Black woman to have trained in thoracic surgery and certified in 1986.[13] As of 2017, however, there were only 6 female African American CT surgeons practicing in the United States.[14]

The history of Latin American CT surgeons was presented at the 2017 STS/European Association for Cardiothoracic Surgery Latin America Cardiovascular Surgery Conference.[15] Highlights included recognizing Dr Manuel Carbonell Salazar as the first surgeon to perform patent ductus arteriosus closures in Cuba in 1941; Drs Pedro Uribe and Svante Tornvall performing a mitral commissurotomy in Chile in 1950; and Dr Marino performing a mitral valvotomy in 1963 as well as the first heart transplant in Peru in 1972. It was also noted that following the development of cardiopulmonary bypass (CPB), the first open-heart surgery in Mexico was performed on an 8-year-old child with an atrial septal defect by Drs Raul Baz Iglesias, Jose Roberto Monroy, and Marcel Garcia Cornejo; and Dr Hugo Fellipozzi performed the first cardiac surgery on CPB in Brazil in 1956.

Latin surgeons who came to and left a lasting impression in the United States include Drs Favaloro, Castaneda, Bastista, Del Nido, among others. Dr Rene Geronimo Favaloro (1923–2000)

was born in Argentina and upon completion of medical school traveled to the Cleveland Clinic to work with Drs Donald B Effner and F Mason Sones. He is known for exploring the possibility of using saphenous vein to bypass diseased segments of a coronary artery circa 1967 and standardized the use of this technique.[16] Dr Aldo R Castaneda (1920–2020) was born in Italy, and after surviving World War II finished college and left Europe for Guatemala to study medicine. His graduation thesis was entitled "Open Heart Surgery: an Experimental Study" and his laboratory research represented the first attempts at open heart surgery in Central America. After completing residency and staying on as faculty at the University of Minnesota, Dr Castaneda was recruited to be the chief of the congenital heart surgery program at Boston Children's Hospital. He is the father of the collaborative and multidisciplinary congenital heart surgery unit and pioneered neonatal and early corrective surgery for complex congenital heart disease. He also developed a fully functioning and independent congenital heart surgery program in Guatemala and was the first Latin president of the AATS.[17] Jose Felix Patino Restrepo (1927–2020) was a Yale School of Medicine graduate (1952), where he also completed his general and CT surgery training. On completing surgical training, Dr Patino returned to Columbia where he was the head of the Department of Surgery at University Hospital of La Samaritana, was the National Minister of Health, and founded Universidad de los Andes School of Medicine, which he modeled after Yale.[18] Dr Randas J Vilela Batista (1947-) from Brazil trained in the United States, Canada, England, and France before returning home in 1983. He is known for several cardiac surgical techniques, including the "Batista procedure," or ventricular remodeling for heart failure.[19] Dr Ivan F Gonzalez-Cancel was the first surgeon to perform a heart transplant in Puerto Rico in 1999. Dr Pedro J del Nido (born in Chile), who trained in CT surgery at the University of Toronto and at the Hospital for Sick Children as a congenital heart surgeon, is known for his work on myocardial energetics and cardioplegia and extracorporeal life support in children.[20] He is currently the Chief of Cardiac Surgery at Boston Children's Hospital and was the 94th president of the AATS.

CURRENT ASSESSMENT OF THE CT WORKFORCE

Although data on the entire CT surgery workforce are not available, in their study Ortmeyer and colleagues[21] used data from the Association of American Medical Colleges (AAMC) and reported that

17%, 3%, and 5% of CT surgeons in academia were women, Black, and Hispanic, respectively. In the 2020 WTS update, of 176 female respondents, 19% were Asian, 6% Black, and 4% Hispanic. These data on women in CT surgery trended toward increased diversity as compared to the 2012 report.[8] In comparison, 43%, 20%, 4%, and 6% of all clinical faculty in academic medicine are women, Asian, Black, and Hispanic, respectively. In addition, 51%, 18%, 13%, and 6% of the US population are women, Hispanic, Black, and Asian, respectively.[22]

In recognition of the fact that women and URM CT surgeons have experiences and needs unique from nonminoritized CT surgeons, the STS sponsored diversity and gender bias surveys in collaboration with the STS Diversity Task Force and WTS. The results of both surveys were reported in several articles published by both entities.[23–25] Gender bias was noted as being pervasive in the discipline and being subjected to sexual harassment was reported by 80% of female attendings and 90% of female trainees.[24,25] Although the authors acknowledge that the response rate to their survey was low, Erhunmwunsee and colleagues[23] reported that 70% of women (compared to 25% men), 83% of Black, and 39% of Asian CT surgeons (compared to 27% White/Caucasian) felt they had been unfairly treated based on their gender or race. More disconcerting were quotes noted in Diversity Task Force's report on myths, barriers, and strategies on improving diversity[26]:

> [The STS] doesn't need to [address diversity] and this should not even be on the radar of things to be done.

> I do not believe barriers exist. This myth of the necessity of diversity and inclusiveness is political correctness on steroids.

> There are no barriers. None of the above are important!

These quotes from survey respondents indicated that members of our discipline did not see a need for focusing on diversity and inclusion. Similarly, with regards to gender bias, responses from male CT surgeons diverged vastly from responses from female CT surgeons, indicating that most of the (male) surgeons did not even recognize the existence of the biased work environment.[24] These reports confirmed that women, Asian, Black, and Hispanic CT surgeons were in the minority but also that these underrepresented surgeons perceived a hostile work environment.

Representation and Leadership

The racial diversity and progression of minorities to leadership in academic surgery was recently studied, whereupon AAMC census data over a 6-year period were examined.[27] Of more than 15,000 surgical faculty diversity was similar at the instructor level but noted to have increased among associate professors over the study period (26.9% in 2013 to 31.9% in 2019). Representation from Asians increased and was the driver of this increase in diversity at the associate professor level (16.9% in 2013 to 20.5% in 2019). Black surgical faculty remain underrepresented at all levels with a slight improvement at the instructor (2.9% in 2013 to 4.5% in 2019) and associate professor (2.7% in 2013 to 3.7% in 2019) levels. Hispanic faculty remain underrepresented at all levels and remained stable (5.6% instructors, 6.8% assistant professors, and 5.1% associate professors in 2019). There was a more favorable trend with regards to growth for Black and Hispanic women compared with Black and Hispanic men, whereas among Asian surgical faculty, the trend was more favorable for men than women. At the full professor level, Asian faculty had the greatest increase (9.2% in 2013 to 13.3% in 2019) with minimal change among Black (2.3% vs 2.7%) and Hispanic (4.0% vs 4.4%) faculty. There was an increase in diversity among surgical department Chairs (19.0% in 2013%–22.6% in 2019), with 12.4%, 5.3%, and 3.4% of Chairs being Asian, Hispanic, and Black, respectively. By 2019, only one Black woman and one Hispanic woman had ascended to Chair.

With the increase in awareness of the importance of diversity, studies on the representation of women at national CT surgery organization meetings have ensued. Olive and colleagues reported that in 2018, 12.9% and 7.9% of presenting and senior authors were women, and that these numbers were similar compared to 3 years prior.[28] In their study, Shemanski and colleagues found that of 3662 session leaders (moderators, panelists, invited discussants) across 20 different CT surgery professional organization annual meetings from 2015 to 2019, 13.1% were women. The proportion of women session leaders trended positively over time from 9.6% in 2015 to 15.9% in 2019 ($P = .001$). However, the increase in female session leaders over time was significant only in General Thoracic sessions and not in Adult Cardiac or Congenital sessions. Lastly, 57.4% of the sessions consisted of all-male session leadership.[29] The Annals of Thoracic Surgery editorial board has had an increase in female members (15.7% in 2018) and more women are holding nominated STS leadership positions (12.3% in 2018).[28]

In the 2021 to 2022 academic year, the STS board of directors consists of 4 (18.2%) women, 3 (13.6%) Asian, and 1 (4.5%) Black CT surgeon. The STS has had one Black past president (Dr Robert SD Higgins) and one female past president (Dr Carolyn E Reed) who was elected posthumously. On the AATS board of directors reside 2 women (12.5%), 3 Asian (18.8%), and 1 Black (6.2%) CT surgeon. The first female president (Dr Yolanda L Colson) will be residing this upcoming year and 2 Latin CT surgeons (Drs Aldo R Castaneda and Pedro J del Nido) have been past presidents. Studies suggest that for a minority group to have influence in the decisions of a committee, a presence of at least 25% is required.[30] CT surgery has yet to reach the 25% threshold in diversity in representation or leadership.

CONSIDERATIONS AND FUTURE DIRECTIONS
Barriers to Increasing Diversity in CT

Several barriers remain as obstacles to achieving increased diversity and equity. First and foremost, there are myths revolving around the goal of diversity. In their study, Backhus and colleagues[26] reported that 21% of respondents to the STS Diversity Task Force survey expressed concerns that diversity was about exclusivity and reverse discrimination. Respondents also expressed concerns that diversity was about lowering standards (12%) and that it does not support meritocracy (18%). Most concerning was that 15% of responses reflected beliefs that disparities did not exist. Until we, as a profession and culture, acknowledge that inequities based on race and gender among us exist, we cannot move forward toward correcting the imbalance within our discipline. Moreover, it cannot be emphasized enough that proponents of diversity, above all else, insist on changes and improvements being based on merit and accomplishments. Advancing those who are ill-equipped and unprepared would only be to the demise of our profession and hinder the goal of increasing diversity.

The pipeline is often cited as a barrier toward increased diversity. In reality, women have been matriculating into medical school regularly and in 2017, more women matriculated into medical school than men. Despite this fact, however, only 24% of current CT surgical trainees, 17% of CT surgeons in academia, and 7% of CT surgeons in the United States are women. Similarly, even though 7.3% and 6.5% of current medical graduates are Black and Hispanic, these racial groups only represent 3% and 5% of CT surgical faculty, respectively. The diversity in medical school remains greater than the diversity in CT surgery, suggesting that there are cultural barriers within our profession that stunts the successful recruitment of diverse candidates to our field. These cultural barriers include implicit biases as well as the lack of an inclusive environment. Moreover, studies suggest that for an individual to succeed in their careers having mentors and sponsors is crucial. Although having same-gender or same-race mentors is not required, trainees have expressed a preference for and increased comfort with same-gender mentors.[31,32] Similarly, data suggest that it is difficult for an underrepresented in medicine (UIM) medical student to envision themselves pursuing a career within a specialty in the paucity of same gender/race faculty in that field.

Programs/Efforts that Promote Diversity in the Workforce

To effect sustainable change and to improve diversity in our specialty, a systematic, multidisciplinary, and programmatic approach is necessary. Realistic goals need to be established. However, first and foremost, unyielding endorsement and resources from leadership is mandatory. Efforts must be multilevel and result in change at every step of progression in a physician's career. Colleges and medical schools should be applauded for their recognition of the importance of DEI and their national efforts in recruitment, a topic that is beyond the scope of this article. As a discipline, we ought to follow suit with deliberate efforts toward increasing DEI in CT surgery residency and fellowship training. These efforts should continue through early and midcareer development through progression toward levels of leadership and late career.

Ortmeyer and colleagues[33] outlined a checklist for increasing diversity in CT surgery training programs. In their literature review of articles on "diversity," "inclusion," "surgery," and "thoracic surgery," the authors identified themes that resulted in successful DEI initiatives and aptly developed an acronym checklist toward DEI—GOALS. The first letter identifies the first step toward change as the establishment of succinct and actionable **g**oals—developing a mission statement, ascertaining the scope of existing disparities, setting metrics for monitoring progress. The second letter represents the need for leadership support for an **o**rganizational change led from the top down. In this, the creation of task forces and the empowerment of these task forces to act is necessary. In addition, leadership ought to provide resources (in the form of recognition,

administrative and salary support, promotion) for these task forces to achieve named goals. **A**dvocacy and support structures for UIM lend toward recruitment efforts as well as retention. These efforts include involvement in local and national UIM organizations, the establishment of formal mentorship programs, training faculty to recognize discrimination, harassment and bias, and creating safe spaces and support groups for UIM. Increasing resident and faculty diversity **l**iteracy—implicit bias training, delineate the effects of discrimination and microaggression, teach use of inclusive language, emphasize the role and importance of diversity in health care—through educational programs should be mandatory for all. Lastly, and most importantly, **s**ustainability of DEI initiatives with monitoring of progress, reassessment and revision of goals is paramount.

Similarly, these GOALS can be applied to DEI initiatives following CT surgery training. In their statement on diversity and inclusion in CT surgery, the STS Diversity Task Force categorized efforts into multiple spheres of influence.[3] Focusing on the CT surgery community level, several professional organizations have endorsed and enacted initiatives to advocate for increased diversity. WTS provides a social network to support women in the discipline and has been successful in developing several scholarships to facilitate student-faculty mentorship as well as early and midcareer development. The AATS has dedicated leadership development courses to women (2018) and UIM (2021) in CT surgery. The STS has named goals of diversity and with those goals has dedicated funding toward DEI initiatives, named an entire symposium focused on DEI during each annual meeting (the Vivien Thomas Lecture), and has mandates with respect to the representation of UIM as invited moderators, panelists, or discussants.

As a discipline and as individuals, we can further advocate for DEI and support our UIM colleagues by being deliberate in selecting faculty for invited lectureships, committee members, and chairs, and as guest editors for medical journals. These mentoring actions assist in faculty development and career progression. Although mentorship is important, studies have shown that sponsorship is the key ingredient to attaining leadership positions.[34] As such, we should be deliberate in sponsoring UIM and providing them with opportunities they would otherwise not be privy to. By being supportive and methodical in assuring representation from all minority groups, we foster inclusion and create an environment whereupon all can be successful.

SUMMARY

Although colleges and medical schools have made strides in increasing the diversity among student populations, CT surgery remains predominantly male and White with limited women, Black, and Hispanic surgeons. Fostering diversity benefits the work culture, fosters innovation, and most importantly, improves patient care. To increase the diversity of our discipline, CT surgery and its leaders ought to establish clear DEI goals, foster inclusion, and be deliberate in instituting plans to attain these goals.

DISCLOSURE

Ceppa (AstraZeneca [consultant], Medtronic [consultant]).

ACKNOWLEDGMENTS

The authors would like to thank L Erhunmwunswee, N Villamizar, and D Avella for reviewing sections of this article.

REFERENCES

1. Erkmen CP, Ortmeyer KA, Cooke DT. Diversity in cardiothoracic surgery: beyond a "Gender/Color-Blind" approach. Ann Thorac Surg 2021. S0003-4975(21)00991-7.
2. Backhus LM, Fann BE, Hui DS, et al. Culture of safety and gender inclusion in cardiothoracic surgery. Ann Thorac Surg 2018;106(4):951–8.
3. Erkmen CP, Ortmeyer KA, Pelletier GJ, et al. An approach to diversity and inclusion in cardiothoracic surgery. Ann Thorac Surg 2021;111(3):747–52.
4. Cooke DT, Olive J, Godoy L, et al. The importance of a diverse specialty: introducing the sts workforce on diversity and inclusion. Ann Thorac Surg 2019; 108(4):1000–5.
5. Available at: https://www.aats.org/aatsimis/AATSWeb/Association/About/Diversity_Inclusion_and_Equity_Statement.aspx. Accessed June 21, 2021.
6. Antonoff MB, David EA, Donington JS, et al. Women in thoracic surgery: 30 years of history. Ann Thorac Surg 2016;101(1):399–409.
7. Preventza O, Backhus L. US women in thoracic surgery: reflections on the past and opportunities for the future. J Thorac Dis 2021;13(1):473–9.
8. Ceppa DP, Antonoff MB, Tong BC, et al. 2020 Women in Thoracic Surgery update on the status of women in cardiothoracic surgery. Ann Thorac Surg 2021. [E-pub ahead of print].
9. Dresler CM, Padgett DL, MacKinnon SE, et al. Experiences of women in cardiothoracic surgery. A gender comparison. Arch Surg 1996;131(11): 1128–34 [Discussion 1135].
10. Donington JS, Litle VR, Sesti J, et al. The WTS report on the current status of women in cardiothoracic surgery. Ann Thorac Surg 2012;94(2):452–8 [Discussion 458–9].
11. Available at: https://www.heart.org/en/news/2020/02/21/9-african-american-pioneers-in-medicine. Accessed May 11, 2021.
12. McCabe K. Available at: https://www.washingtonian.com/2020/06/19/the-remarkable-story-of-vivien-thomas-the-black-man-who-helped-invent-heart-surgery/. Accessed May 11, 2021.
13. Available at: https://med.stanford.edu/ctsurgery/about-the-department/news/2021/ct-surgery-celebrating-black-history-month.html. Accessed May 11, 2021.
14. Okereke I. Commentary: we need diversity in cardiothoracic surgery. J Thorac Cardiovasc Surg 2020. [E-pub ahead of print].
15. Available at: https://www.sts.org/sites/default/files/documents/Latin_America_2017/Friday_9-22-2017/1015_Fri_History%20CV%20Surgery_Jatene.pdf. Accessed May 19, 2021.
16. Available at: https://en.wikipedia.org/wiki/Ren%C3%A9_Favaloro. Accessed June 4, 2021.
17. Available at: https://www.aats.org/aatsimis/AATSWeb/Foundation/Programs/Programs/Aldo_R._Castaneda/Honoring_Aldo_R_Castaneda.aspx. Accessed June 11, 2021.
18. Available at: https://medicine.yale.edu/news-article/colombias-top-doctor-yale-trained-jose-felix-patino-dies/. Accessed June 1, 2021.
19. Available at: https://www.ctsnet.org/article/randas-j-vilela-batista-md. Accessed June 4, 2021.
20. Spratt JR, Guleserian KJ, Shumway SJ. Historical perspectives of The American Association for Thoracic Surgery: Pedro J. del Nido. J Thorac Cardiovasc Surg 2017;153(2):225–7.
21. Ortmeyer KA, Raman V, Tiko-Okoye C, et al. Women and minorities underrepresented in academic cardiothoracic surgery: it's time for next steps. Ann Thorac Surg 2020. [E-pub ahead of print].
22. Available at: https://www.census.gov/quickfacts/fact/table/US/PST045219. Accessed May 19, 2021.
23. Erhunmwunsee L, Backhus LM, Godoy L, et al. Report from the workforce on diversity and inclusion-the society of thoracic surgeons members' bias experiences. Ann Thorac Surg 2019;108(5): 1287–91.
24. Ceppa DP, Dolejs SC, Boden N, et al. Gender bias and its negative impact on cardiothoracic surgery. Ann Thorac Surg 2020;109(1):14–7.
25. Ceppa DP, Dolejs SC, Boden N, et al. Sexual harassment and cardiothoracic surgery: #UsToo? Ann Thorac Surg 2020;109(4):1283–8.

26. Backhus LM, Kpodonu J, Romano JC, et al. An exploration of myths, barriers, and strategies for improving diversity among STS Members. Ann Thorac Surg 2019;108(6):1617–24.

27. Riner AN, Herremans KM, Neal DW, et al. Diversification of academic surgery, its leadership, and the importance of intersectionality. JAMA Surg 2021. [E-pub ahead of print].

28. Olive JK, Preventza OA, Blackmon SH, et al. Representation of women in the society of thoracic surgeons authorship and leadership positions. Ann Thorac Surg 2020;109(5):1598–604.

29. Shemanski KA, Ding L, Kim AW, et al. Gender representation among leadership at national and regional cardiothoracic surgery organizational annual meetings. J Thorac Cardiovasc Surg 2021;161(3):733–44.

30. Centola D, Becker J, Brackbill D, et al. Experimental evidence for tipping points in social convention. Science 2018;360(6393):1116–9.

31. Luc JGY, Stamp NL, Antonoff MB. Social media in the mentorship and networking of physicians: Important role for women in surgical specialties. Am J Surg 2018;215(4):752–60.

32. Bettis J, Thrush CR, Slotcavage RL, et al. What makes them different? An exploration of mentoring for female faculty, residents, and medical students pursuing a career in surgery. Am J Surg 2019;218(4):767–71.

33. Ortmeyer KA, Raman V, Tiko-Okoye CS, et al. Goals, organizational change, advocacy, diversity literacy, and sustainability: a checklist for diversity in cardiothoracic surgery training programs. J Thorac Cardiovasc Surg 2020. [E-pub ahead of print].

34. Carter NM. Mentoring: necessary but insufficient for advancement 2010. Available at: https://wwwcatalystorg/wp-content/uploads/2019/01/Mentoring_Necessary_But_Insufficient_for_Advancement_Final_120610pdf. Accessed September 2, 2020.

Moving?

Make sure your subscription moves with you!

To notify us of your new address, find your **Clinics Account Number** (located on your mailing label above your name), and contact customer service at:

Email: journalscustomerservice-usa@elsevier.com

800-654-2452 (subscribers in the U.S. & Canada)
314-447-8871 (subscribers outside of the U.S. & Canada)

Fax number: 314-447-8029

Elsevier Health Sciences Division
Subscription Customer Service
3251 Riverport Lane
Maryland Heights, MO 63043

ELSEVIER